Praise for *Why Does It Hurt?*

I've been frustrated too many times to count with
pain descriptions and patterns that don't fit the traditional dermatomes
we all learned in medical school. FDM offers explanations for complex
pain questions that traditional medical teaching doesn't explain. It's
revolutionized my practice!

Grayson T. Westfall, MD, Director 1st care,
Tanana Valley Clinic, Fairbanks, Alaska

FDM is one of the greatest tools I have, especially for
patients who want to go back and participate in the sports
that they were injured in.

Juan F. Acosta, DO, MS, FACOEP-D
Assistant Dean of Postgraduate Medical Education
Associate Professor, Department of Osteopathic Principles and Practice
Pacific Northwest University of Health Sciences
College of Osteopathic Medicine

Since adding FDM to my hands-on treatments I've been able to accurately
diagnose and treat conditions that may have escaped traditional allopathic
and osteopathic approaches.

Drew Lewis, DO, Diplomat AOBPM&R, FAAPM&R,
Board Certified in Physical Medicine and Rehabilitation
Assistant Professor, Osteopathic Manual Medicine Department
Des Moines University

Why Does It Hurt?

The Fascial Distortion Model:
A new paradigm for pain relief and restored movement

TODD A. CAPISTRANT, DO, MHA.
With Steve LeBeau

BEAVER'S
POND
PRESS

Edited by Alicia Ester

ISBN 13: 978-1-59298-941-6

Library of Congress Catalog Number: 2014903082

Printed in the United States of America

Second Printing: 2015

19 18 17 16 15   6 5 4 3 2

Artwork by Brianna Reagan Art, © 2013
Cover and interior design by James Monroe Design, LLC.

Beaver's Pond Press, Inc.
7108 Ohms Lane
Edina, MN 55439–2129
(952) 829-8818
www.BeaversPondPress.com

BEAVER'S
POND
PRESS

To order, visit ItascaBooks.com
or call (800) 901-3480. Reseller discounts available.

Dedication

I would like to dedicate this book to the patients:
past, present, and future. To the ups and downs in the
treatment and relief of your pain. Thank you for
guiding me on this journey.

Contents

Introduction

It sounds like a miracle, but it's not.

A basketball player sprains his ankle during the first half of a game. A physician with a special technique digs into that ankle with his thumb for about a minute. The injured player stands up. The sprain is gone. He plays the entire second half without pain and his team wins the game. No crutches, no medication, no ice. Nothing but net.

The pain in an elderly lady's back is so severe, she walks stooped over at a forty-five-degree angle. She's been this way for as long as anyone can remember. She requires a cane to walk. A physician with special skills digs into certain points in her back with his thumb for a couple of minutes. The woman stands up straight and is pain-free for the first time in years. She feels so good she goes out the door and walks for three miles. Without her cane.

A young physician attending a medical conference is uncomfortable because of the deep ache in his elbows. He's had tennis elbow in both arms for two years and nothing has worked. Not painkillers. Not physical therapy. Nothing. A couple of physicians with special skills dig their thumbs into his elbows for a minute or two. When he gets up the next morning, he realizes his pain is gone.

That physician with the sore arms was me. Those colleagues grabbing my arms were introducing me in a very visceral way to a new approach called the Fascial Distortion Model, or FDM for short. I learned that it was more than a technique; it was a whole new approach to how the body works. When they fixed my arms, they sent my medical career into a new direction.

No, it's not a miracle. It only seems like one because this simple solution to all kinds of musculoskeletal pain and dysfunction is virtually unheard of. The secret is fascia (pronounced **fash**-*uh*)—understanding how fascia works, how it wraps and interconnects every cell in your body, and how to manipulate it when it gets distorted.

What's the catch? Well, it can hurt quite a bit when physicians dig their thumbs into you. But it's a good pain. It's like pulling out a sliver; it hurts while they're doing it, but when they're done, it feels so good. While some of the most common distortions are painful when treated, not all distortions require a painful treatment to be corrected.

Any special medications? No.

Any fancy high-priced technology? Not really. Only my fingernail clippers. I have to keep my thumbnails pretty short so I don't cut anybody when I'm working my thumb into their distorted fascia.

So what is fascia, anyway?

Fascia is that fibrous silvery tissue, almost like a spider web, that wraps all your muscles, all your organs, your bones, your ligaments, everything. You've seen it whenever you've pulled the skin off a piece of chicken or other meat. It used to be that fascia was only considered valuable as a type of packing material for our body, but that simplistic view is changing. Now research into the multiple functions of fascia is one of the frontiers of medical science. It is the view of the FDM that fascia is essential for all bodily movements in the musculoskeletal structure. It is a living flexible interface between all of our moving parts that allows them to slide and glide past each other without friction. But when fascia gets distorted—wrinkled, tangled, torn, whatever—then movement becomes limited or impossible. Plus it becomes painful, because fascia is loaded with nerve cells. So when a sprained ankle hurts and you can't put weight on it, in most cases it's not a torn muscle or a stretched ligament that takes six weeks to heal; the problem is that the fascia in your ankle has been altered—so you simply rearrange it with your thumb. It's really not that hard; you just have to have been introduced to this different way of looking at pain. The essential fact about fascia is that it was made to move, and the more it moves, the healthier it is. The same is true for you as a person. The more you move, the healthier you will be. My job is to get people moving again.

Pain

One of the top reasons that people go to see a doctor is pain, and the most prevalent form is musculoskeletal pain.[1] I'm willing to bet that the number one reason for repeat medical visits is chronic pain. We have a lot of aches and pains in our bodies that conventional medicine does not know how to fix. Instead, medicine has developed habitual ways to deal with various complaints about musculoskeletal pain, even though quite often the treatments are not successful. So people with chronic pain keep receiving expensive tests, continue physical therapy, and get prescription after prescription of narcotic medications. Chronic pain is an expensive issue, costing billions each year.

The purpose of this book is to tell you that it doesn't have to be this way. We have learned to successfully treat a variety of common problems more effectively than conventional medicine. I started doing Fascial Distortion Model treatments while I was a primary care physician at a walk-in clinic. I figure that about a third of the patients I treated responded successfully to traditional osteopathic manipulation, about a third responded somewhat well, and about a third did not respond to manipulation at all. But now the vast majority of my patients find significant relief from their pain and stiffness. I feel that I am doing a good thing for thousands of people, and now I want to spread the word.

This book is for chronic pain sufferers who haven't found a solution. It is for athletes, dancers, soldiers, and others who need the full use of their bodies for their livelihoods. This is for those active people who do not want to walk around on crutches for six weeks because of a sprained ankle. This book is also for physicians who want to learn a new way of looking at human physiology to help diagnose and treat their patients. This book is for physical therapists, yoga instructors, students of anatomy, and anyone else who wants to learn about why our bodies move the way they do.

There's one more special group of people that I want to read this book: my current and future patients. My technique is simple, but it takes some time to explain the philosophy behind it. When I see patients, I may spend fifteen minutes telling them what a fascial distortion is, how fascia works, and what I will be doing for and to them. But the treatment itself may only take thirty seconds. I hope this book will provide the foundation to help them understand what is causing their pain and limited movement.

Key Concept: Knowledge Begins with the Patient

One of the absolute key components of the Fascial Distortion Model is the idea that the patient is the expert. The patient will tell us and show us exactly what is wrong if we physicians just stop and listen to what they are saying. Over and over in medical training, this idea is taught to us. In the FDM the patient will truly guide us to the diagnosis, location, and treatments that are needed to provide them relief.

You will note that this flow of knowledge is exactly the opposite of the contemporary scientific hierarchy's, which holds that knowledge flows from the top down. A series of million dollar research studies explore a new treatment, and after years (often one or two decades[2]) that knowledge trickles down to the practitioners through journal articles and continuing education courses. That's the established pattern now, though it wasn't always that way.

The grassroots flow of knowledge from the patients up is generally disregarded by the powers that be as "mere anecdotal reports." In other words, we FDM practitioners have an uphill battle in our effort to win broad acceptance for the FDM. We are bucking the trend.

But that's okay, because I'm from a tradition of bucking the trend. I'm an osteopathic physician, a crosscurrent within mainstream medicine. The initials *DO* follow our name. They stand for "doctor of osteopathy." We get all the training of a conventional medical doctor, and in a clinic or an emergency room, you often cannot tell us apart. We have a different philosophy than the traditional MD, however, and learn manipulative skills, similar to what a chiropractor might do but often with a wider array of techniques and styles. We approach the human body and mind as an interconnected whole; we were holistic before it was cool. That's why we trust a patient's intuitive knowledge of what is bothering him or her.

The founder of the FDM was a DO, Dr. Stephen Typaldos. He came across the important functions of fascia while listening to a patient who had a strong intuition about how to rid herself of back pain. She was the expert, and she just happened to find a good listener. He combined his theoretical knowledge of physiology with this intuition from his patient, and concluded that the source of her pain was distorted fascia. Manipulating fascia with his thumb straightened it out and brought pain relief. He developed that insight into the FDM, which classifies six main types of fascial distortions. It is by listening to patients' descriptions of their pain and by watching their body language that we figure out which distortion is the source of their pain.

Some day we will have our million dollar studies to validate our knowledge in the eyes of the scientific establishment, but for now we FDM practitioners feel validated every time a patient is freed from pain, every time a hockey player can get back on the ice, and every time a soldier can rejoin his unit. I have treated thousands of patients, and I am convinced that they have led us in the right direction, and helped us uncover a basic new truth about how our bodies work.

Chapter Previews

Chapter One tells the story of the Fascial Distortion Model's discovery and development, and how I came to be involved. The foundation and the application of the FDM emphasize the importance of the patient as the initiator and guide for the treatments. The chapter will also give a fuller explanation of the origin of osteopathy and its inclusion in the medical mainstream early in the twentieth century. I cannot emphasize enough that FDM is not simply a technique or a skill; it is a whole new perspective on how the body operates as a functional unit. It is this understanding that allows us to apply all styles of manipulation techniques in the FDM.

Chapter Two explains fascia, the mystery behind the "miracle." Special emphasis is given to its role in holding the structure of the body together, allowing fluent movement, and conveying pain. You will learn about an architectural concept developed by R. Buckminster Fuller, the creator of the geodesic dome and other out-of-the box inventions. This concept is called *tensegrity*, the ability of an integrated structure to be held together with flexible components that exert tension on rigid components. In a small model you can show tensegrity with a structure of rubber bands and sticks. In the body it becomes *bio*tensegrity, and on a grand scale the rigid elements are bones and the flexible tension is supplied by fascia, which is also linked to the muscles and ligaments. Perhaps the most profound discovery is that some disabling injuries are *only* fascial problems, and can be fixed instantly as long as you have that knowledge (and a strong thumb and a willing patient).

Chapter Three details the nature of each of the six kinds of distortions in the FDM. Some are much more common than others, and they often occur in combination. Sometimes a distortion takes hold, and causes others to arise. An important clue for understanding many instances of chronic musculoskeletal pain is that some distortions are more or less permanent until treated. All of the painkillers in the world will not make them go away. These labels will sound like a foreign language, but they comprise the standard vocabulary of the FDM. It's time to start getting used to their names:

1. Triggerband (TB)

2. Herniated Triggerpoint (HTP)

3. Continuum Distortion (CD)

4. Folding Distortion (FD)

5. Cylinder Distortion (CyD)

6. Tectonic Fixation (TF)

Chapter Four brings case studies of the FDM as applied to some common complaints that I deal with in my practice. I am constantly amazed by several things when treating my patients. First, I am astounded by how long many have endured their particular maladies, usually receiving years of expensive medical treatments and medicines with no lasting results. Second, I am often impressed that success is the result of staying in the model and listening to the patients. Finally, I am always touched by the profound relief and joy that my patients express after a successful treatment. They may refer to me as "Doctor Torture" because of the pain incurred during treatment, but they are thrilled to regain the freedom to move and the freedom from pain. Here are some of the standard ailments I deal with regularly:

- Back pain
- Ankle pain
- Neck pain
- Shoulder pain
- Rib pain
- Headaches
- Pelvic pain
- Abdominal pain
- Pain following breast cancer surgery and other surgery
- Flank pain consistent with kidney stone pain

Chapter Five has stories of the FDM as applied to athletes and other high-performing individuals, such as dancers and soldiers. These people are more likely to sustain injuries because of their intense activities, and they are especially more likely to feel intensely frustrated when injuries put them on the sidelines. These are highly competitive people who are driven to excel. As a result, I see a wide range of emotional response when they finally achieve relief from disabling injuries. I've seen an emotional catharsis that entailed hours of crying, and I've faced anger from people who were mad that such a simple fix wasn't applied much earlier. Here are some of their injuries and ailments:

- Shoulder pain

- Thigh pain

- Knee pain

- Sprained ankles

- Wrist pain

Chapter Six addresses a number of frequently asked questions about FDM. People wonder how they can prepare for treatments and what they should do afterward. I tell them to stay in touch with their pain and help me track it down. Show me how and where it hurts. And after treatment, as always, the best thing is to keep moving. Fascia is made to move. Others wonder how the FDM relates to other methods of treatment, from acupuncture to Rolfing (Structural Integration). For the most part, various other methodologies are compatible or even complementary. Some focus on the fascia and even have similar philosophies as to how this tissue functions within the body. Often these modalities have narrowed their view to one function of the fascia that can be explained by one of our distortions. The FDM is a more complete theory as to the complex function of fascia.

Chapter Seven outlines our progress toward gaining acceptance of the FDM in the mainstream medical community, and why I think it should be part of all medical training. I have no doubt that practitioners trained in the FDM should be available for every sports team, every school, and every military base. We should have the FDM available in our emergency rooms. I expound on the financial savings we could have if the health-care system instituted the FDM instead of insisting on expensive alternatives that don't work for many patients. This chapter also provides an update on our progress entering the curriculum of osteopathic medical schools.

My goal is for you to understand that the Fascial Distortion Model is not simply a technique, but a whole new way of approaching the human body and its musculoskeletal ailments. FDM's biggest lesson is that people should stay active. FDM's most important expert is the patient.

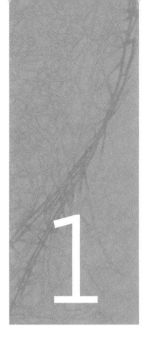

The Discovery of the Fascial Distortion Model

Never underestimate the intelligence of your body as a guide toward better health. It was a determined patient who led to the discovery of the Fascial Distortion Model. In 1991, Dr. Stephen Typaldos, DO, had three patients in a row with nearly identical back pain. All three were women. The first one described a pain that started in her mid-back between the spine and the shoulder blades and then went up the neck toward the ear. Dr. Typaldos was baffled. He tried some of the usual osteopathic manipulation that he frequently used, but she received little relief. He told her there was little more he could do and sent her away with a prescription. He was a bit surprised when the second woman had the same complaint, but he also sent her away with a prescription— and again little relief. The third patient described the pain exactly the same way, but she had a different attitude. She would not listen when he said he couldn't help her.

"I know you can fix this," she insisted.

"But," Dr. Typaldos replied, "I don't know what this is."

"I know you can fix this. You need to push on it," she said.

"It? What is *it*? What are you talking about?"

To his great credit, Dr. Typaldos decided that he needed to give some thought to this right away, so he asked her to

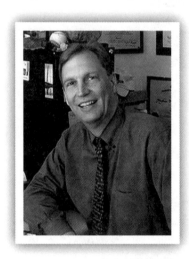

wait while he went to his office to ponder the problem. Fate had dealt him a puzzle, and—in the form of the third patient—insisted that he solve it. Physicians do not often have the opportunity to go sit in their office to think, because there are always more patients to see, forms to complete, or students to teach. But he sat and thought, reaching way back into his mind as he contemplated what to do. Finally he concluded, "I'm going to listen to the patient, and she is going to tell me what to do."

He came back into the room and she said, "I want you to push on it."

"Okay, I'll do whatever you say."

She said, "That's it! Push harder!"

"What is *it*?"

"Push harder! Yes, you are on it, follow it."

"What is she talking about?" Dr. Typaldos wondered, but he kept pushing as hard as he could along the painful spot, and he followed it up right to the base of the lower neck near the mastoid, just below the ear.

When he was done the patient jumped up and said, "I knew it! You are the only one who could do it. I'm fine. It's gone! It is all better!"

And then Dr. Typaldos sat down again, to reflect on what had just happened. Over the next few years he continued to be guided by his patients as they described their pain. He paid close attention to both the words they used and the body language they demonstrated, including how they used their hands and fingers to point out the pain. He soon realized that the mysterious "it" was distorted fascia. Fascia is the thin fibrous membrane that is wrapped around every cell of a body, including groups of muscle fibers and other tissues. The solution to his patients' pain was to manipulate the distorted fascia back into place with his hands. He named his new approach the Fascial Distortion Model (FDM), and created the terminology and procedures that are now used by practitioners of FDM around the world.[3]

Osteopathy

It is no coincidence that the founder of the Fascial Distortion Model was an osteopathic physician, a medical practitioner who has all the training of an MD, but with additional training in osteopathic manipulation and a different philosophy of healing. Osteopathic physicians learn a holistic philosophy that emphasizes promoting health rather than simply fighting disease. It is as if they look at their patients through a different lens and see different things. Picture the Nicolas Cage character in *National Treasure*, who uses spectacles with multiple lenses to look at the reverse side of the Declaration of Independence. Every time he changes the lenses, he sees something new. Osteopaths see patients through a different lens.

Osteopathy was developed in the 1870s by Dr. Andrew Taylor Still, a second generation MD who became disenchanted with the orthodox medical practice of the day. The nineteenth century was the Wild West era of medicine in America. No one had yet learned about germs, and quite often surgeries were performed in unsanitary conditions. The standard medicines of the day included arsenic, opium, and cocaine. Antibiotics had not yet been invented. Dr. Still was also very frustrated with the way the medical profession tended to compartmentalize the human body, rather than seeing it function as a whole.

He believed that when a person stays active and his or her body functions symmetrically, the body can prevent illness, and heal itself when illness arises. His emphasis on anatomy comes through in the discipline's name—*osteo* refers to bones, and *pathy* refers to illness. He also realized that the body can fall out of alignment, so he developed a variety of physical manipulations to help straighten out the limbs, spine, and joints. Some of the manipulations are similar to what a chiropractor might do. In fact, the inventor of chiropractic medicine (Daniel David Palmer) was a disenchanted osteopath who wanted to focus on the spine. But Dr. Still wanted to focus on the body as a whole—and the mind and spirit as well. He was an early advocate of the holistic approach. This was the special lens that he created.

Medical schools were unregulated at the turn of the century and there were no universal standards for becoming a physician. It was, "Anything goes, and let the patient beware!" That's why in 1910 the American Medical Association (AMA) sponsored a critical study of medical education in North America. The project was funded by the Carnegie Foundation and headed by Abraham Flexner. *The Flexner Report* was quite influential in ushering in the era of modern medicine. The report recommended that the more than 150 medical schools be reduced to about thirty, and that practices that could not be verified by science should be excluded. Osteopathy was accepted as an option within the field of medicine. Osteopathic medical students would receive the regular medical education as well as training in osteopathic manipulations. Graduates of osteopathic schools would receive a DO certification instead of the standard MD title. Other practices, including chiropractic, homeopathy, and naturopathy were excluded from certified medical schools. The AMA defines an osteopathic physician as a fully licensed and practicing physician who has the additional skills of manipulation. The focus in osteopathy is more on health, and less on disease. Osteopathic physicians try to focus on the interconnectedness of the body, which then plays a role in any diagnosis or assessment.

Today osteopathy continues to be a small but committed field within modern scientific medicine. According to a 2012 census of actively licensed physicians, there are more than 800,000 MDs in the US, but only around 63,000 DOs.[4] Their orientation toward a holistic approach leads more than half of osteopathic physicians to focus on primary care in their training and in the positions they seek, such as family practice, pediatrics, and internal medicine. In contrast, MDs tend toward specialization, with less than 20 percent going into primary care.

In the last ten years, people have started looking for an osteopathic physician because they want that holistic look at the body. While most osteopaths embrace the holistic approach, very few osteopaths use the manipulative skills they learned in their first two years of medical school. After medical school, when they go on rotations and enter residencies, they are most likely to learn from MDs or DOs that don't do much manipulation. It's no surprise then that only 10 to 20 percent of DOs regularly use manipulations as a form of treatment. Fortunately, Dr. Typaldos was one of those who valued manipulation, for otherwise he would have never developed his FDM. Osteopathic physicians comfortable with using manipulation became fertile ground for the spread of the FDM, but some MDs also adopted the model. Typaldos even found enthusiastic followers of his method in such faraway places as Japan, Germany, and Alaska—where I happen to live.

Dr. Capistrant Encounters the Fascial Distortion Model

I shouldn't say I merely *happen* to live in Alaska, because people rarely move here accidentally. Usually they have a reason for coming and mine was that I enjoy dogsledding. It goes without saying that I really like physical activity and being outdoors. When I decided to become a physician, my love of activity drew me toward becoming an osteopath, which is basically a form of medicine based on the body functioning as a whole. The way I see it, motion is health, and symmetrical motion is what we are seeking as osteopathic physicians. When I am trying to help a patient attain health through holistic wellness, the organs are working together. In the musculoskeletal part of osteopathy, I am looking for a symmetrical range of motion—and that will lead to health.

That's the theory, anyway. It works well until you come up with some sort of painful physical ailment that gets in the way of enjoying physical activity. In my case, I developed severe tennis elbow in both arms. The deep aching pain in my elbows made it difficult for me to use my arms because they hurt so much. Sometimes the pain was so bad, it would wake me up at night. I tried everything to fix the ache in my elbows. I went to orthopedists and physical therapists, tried multiple styles of braces, took all kinds of medication, and did anything suggested that might help relieve the pain. I even received several steroid injections. None of these treatments provided me with any lasting relief. This went on for at least two years. The pain had become a focus of my life and I was depressed because of it. I couldn't fully enjoy activities anymore—especially dogsledding.

Throughout my bout with tennis elbow I continued to work at a walk-in clinic in Fairbanks. Like all physicians, I needed to attend continuing medical education (CME) courses to maintain my state license. I decided to attend a CME conference held by the Alaska Osteopathic Medical Association (AKOMA) in Anchorage, a six-hour drive. The drive was an added chore because even holding the steering wheel bothered my elbows.

It turned out that Dr. Typaldos was also planning a two-and-a-half day course on his FDM in Anchorage just before the CME conference. I might have attended his workshop except for two small things: time and money. I could not take the extra time off work nor was I able to afford the registration fee. So, I showed up for the start of the usual CME course and attended some excellent presentations on topics important to my practice. My fellow participants noticed that I was in a fair amount of distress because I was constantly rubbing my arms and really struggling to remain comfortable during the lectures.

During one of the breaks, I was speaking with a few other physicians when the topic of my pain came up. I explained to them how I had been battling tennis elbow for several years. Some of them had attended the FDM workshop, and couldn't hide the excitement in their eyes when they heard about my chronic pain. They became very animated and began jabbering about how they knew what was wrong with me and could fix it. It almost seemed like they were speaking a foreign language: "triggerband," "fascial distortion," "tectonic fixation." I had never heard of the distortions they were speaking about or the different treatments they were suggesting. The model was a completely foreign concept to me. This was particularly disheartening because I really enjoyed performing manipulation and it was an important part of my practice. I felt really out of touch.

Their excitement escalated as they swirled around me. Then, with practically no warning, a couple of them grabbed my arms and told me they were going to "treat" me. They dug their thumbs into the sorest parts of my elbows, causing intense pain. I swear the tears shot several inches out of my eyes. After each bout of elbow torture they would stop and ask, "Where is the pain now?" I could hardly wrap my mind around what they were doing to me, plus the pain kept changing, so I was rather slow to respond. Suddenly I heard a chime indicating that the break was over and they were about to announce the next speaker. My session was done! I had survived the treatment. Thank goodness.

I sat through the remaining lectures with throbbing forearms and elbows. They were tender to the touch. The physicians had encouraged me to apply ice, so I went back to my hotel room and did just as I was instructed. The next morning, as I was getting ready for more lectures, I realized my tennis elbow was gone. For the first time in nearly two years, my elbows did not ache. They were definitely tender to the touch, but the deep aching that often caused me so much discomfort was gone. I was shocked and confused, but also quite happy.

At the first opportunity I told the physicians who had treated me about my relief, and I asked them to explain what they had done. What was the theory behind those treatments? They gave me a quick explanation of the fascial distortions and the FDM, using the same mysterious terminology they had used the day before. I was amazed that after all this time my elbows no longer hurt.

On my six-hour drive from Anchorage back to Fairbanks, I had plenty of time to consider just what had happened. I thought about how much the elbow pain had taken from me. I realized that the pain had prevented me from enjoying my dog team. But now the pain was gone and it was as if I had gotten my regular life back. I still wasn't really clear as to what this FDM was, but I was impressed.

My First Triggerband Treatment

During my next shift at the walk-in clinic, an elderly woman limped into the exam room. She told me she had suffered a deep cut in her leg three years earlier and it was still painful. "When I got hurt my stuff stuck through and I should've had it closed, but I didn't," she said. "I let it scar over. The scab finally fell off and I have been limping ever since." From the size of the scar I saw that she certainly could have used some stitches to close the wound over her right shin. I asked her two of the key questions used when working in the Fascial Distortion Model: "Where is the pain?" and "How does it hurt?" I almost fell off the exam stool when she waved her hand up and down her shin over the scar. I sat staring at what she had just shown me. The body language was exactly what the other physicians had said the patient would show me to indicate a triggerband distortion of fascia.

I pushed the FDM from my mind and tried to focus on what could be wrong with her leg from the perspective of my traditional medical training. I was worried about some form of bone lesion so I ordered an x-ray. That may seem like a stretch, but we often find cancer in patients who have not had regular medical care. I was relieved when the x-ray came back without any changes in the bone. I then repeated the questions of "Where is the pain?" and "How does it hurt?" I was again shocked that she did not change her description. I thought to myself, "This is indeed what they were calling a triggerband."

I decided to ask this nice lady if I could try something. I explained that I had just heard of a newer way of looking at the body that may explain why she was in so much pain. I informed her that I thought she had a triggerband and that the fascia where she had cut herself was twisted, and this was what was causing her pain. I knew the cut had obviously disrupted the fascia under the skin, and this certainty allowed me to accept the FDM concept that fascia can get twisted and distorted. With her kind permission, I took my thumb and followed the three-inch line she had indicated down her shin. She was very tough and tolerated the intense treatment with hardly a sound, even though she was in obvious discomfort. When I finished, she leaped up and ran around the treatment table three times. Her smile was a mile wide and she was no longer limping. She came right up to me and gave me a huge hug. I am pretty sure my jaw was hanging open as she left the exam room laughing and extremely happy. I saw I was not the only one whose years of aching pain could be fixed with a minute or two of simple manipulation.

I had no idea what had just occurred. All I knew was that during the course of my medical school and family practice residency, I had learned nothing that could explain what had happened to this lady. I was dumbstruck. I thought back to the conversations at the conference and remembered that the FDM group was planning another event in Hawaii. I decided I needed to attend.

The New Lens of the Fascial Distortion Model

I started to apply the Fascial Distortion Model to my patients with musculoskeletal pain, whether it was chronic or from a recent injury. Even with my limited knowledge of the FDM, the results were astonishing. My confidence in the model grew as my ability to apply it increased. I worked to understand it more and read Dr. Typaldos' FDM book[5] several times, trying to understand the model as best I could before heading to Hawaii. Unfortunately, Dr. Typaldos passed away in March 2006 and I never had the opportunity to learn directly from him. His students decided to conduct the Hawaii event in spite of his death, and I learned quite a bit from them.

Initially I thought I was learning techniques. I'm sure that's what most people think when they sign up for an FDM course: they're going to learn techniques they can use to treat their patients, just another tool for their kit. In reality, the FDM is so much more. It is a new way of looking at the body. Yes, there are some distinct techniques that can be applied to treat patients. But more importantly, a physician's perspective can change after becoming immersed in the model. I had been given a new set of lenses through which I could view patients' bodies and how they were experiencing pain.

For example, under the lens of conventional medicine, my tennis elbow was inflammation. There was no doubt. Therefore, I received the sort of treatment designed for inflammation, except it didn't work. An MRI of my elbow would have showed there was no inflammation. Nevertheless, the conventional lens dictates that it is inflammation and should be treated as such. Now switch to the osteopathic lens. It looks at the body as a whole and notices how my tennis elbow disrupts my range of activities and reduces my overall health. It does not recommend any different treatments, however. Now switch over to the FDM lens and everything looks totally different. It is not inflammation at all. The problem with my tennis elbow is distorted fascia, something that can be fixed through physical manipulation. This lens provides an entirely different view of the body, especially where musculoskeletal injuries and pain are considered.

One of the things I found before I got into the FDM is that a lot of my manipulation treatments were highly effective on about 33 percent of the people; for another 33 percent, the treatments were effective but issues returned; and for the other 33 percent, the treatments did not work as well as I would have liked. But now when I do the same treatment and incorporate the soft tissue aspects of FDM, the treatments tend to last a lot longer. The more the model worked, the more I followed it, until now—when my practice consists entirely of using the FDM in concert with my osteopathic manipulation.

While attending another FDM course in San Diego, I remember thinking that this was an amazingly powerful tool that should be in the hands of everyone in medicine. However, we were in a terrible situation because there were no teachers of this model in the United States. I decided I needed to work hard and learn enough so that I could teach other people the FDM. I had already helped dozens of people with what seemed like nearly miraculous outcomes. This model could change lives. After all, I was one who had been treated successfully. The new lens had worked for me, and now I wanted to help spread the word.

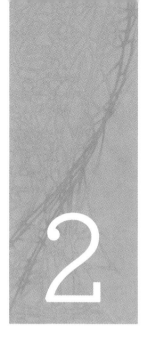

Fascia: The Mystery Behind the Miracle

Everyone is familiar with fascia in some form or other. If you've ever pulled the skin off a piece of chicken, you've seen the shiny, silvery strings that try to keep the skin attached. Our skin is attached the same way, as if we were wearing a bodysuit of fascia that serves to hold our skin onto us. If you pull on the pants leg of your bodysuit, you can feel the tension on your shoulder and other parts of your body. Likewise, if fascia is pulled, its effects can be felt on various other places in your body. But part of the great new understanding of fascia is that it isn't simply two-dimensional like a sheet of plastic. It is three-dimensional. If you pull on it, a tension develops inside the body as well as along the surface. It runs through your insides and it is all connected.

A simple way to illustrate the many layers of fascia is by looking at an orange. You take off the peel and there is layer of fascia holding onto the fruit, but other fascia holds it into sections, and within each section there are the little globules of pulp, also surrounded by fascia. If you go down to the cellular level, you'll find more fascia.

Our current understanding is that fascia is the lattice-work of fibrous tissue that surrounds and connects every cell in our bodies. Like an all-encompassing web, it covers every muscle, bone, and ligament, every organ and nerve within us. Fascia is the matrix that connects all the other tissues and enables us to function as a whole. Scientists and researchers are only beginning to understand the full importance of fascia, because it was ignored for quite a long time. Fascia was originally considered to be just a covering for other body parts, a type of wrapping that had to be torn off to study all the really "important" things like muscles, tendons, bones, and so on. Anatomy students have spent hours removing this tissue in order to see beneath this supposedly inactive layer. As a result, scientists learned a lot about muscles and bones, but not much about fascia. Nearly everyone assumed that fascia was predominantly supportive in nature and had no other function. That's why the tissue was named *fascia*, a Latin word that means a binding or a band, as in a bandage.

An exception to this general disregard of fascia came from the founder of osteopathy, Andrew Taylor Still. In 1899, he devoted a chapter to fascia in his *Philosophy of Oste-opathy*, and declared it a priority for future research:

> [Fascia] being that principle that sheathes,
> permeates, divides, and subdivides every portion
> of all animal bodies; surrounding and penetrating

every muscle and all its fibers—every artery, and every fiber and principle thereunto belonging.

The fascia gives one of, if not the greatest problems to solve as to the part it takes in life and death. It belts each muscle, vein, nerve, and all organs of the body. It is almost a network of nerves, cells, and tubes, running to and from it; it is crossed and filled with, no doubt, millions of nerve centers and fibers to carry on the work of secreting and excreting fluid vital and destructive.

Thus knowledge of the universal extent of the fascia is almost imperative, and is one of the greatest aids to the person who seeks the cause of disease.[6]

Dr. Still was about 100 years ahead of his time because it wasn't until the 1990s that significant numbers of people started taking fascia seriously. Scientific interest is so strong these days that it is considered a kind of Cinderella story. The "Great Ball," as it were, was the International Fascia Research Congress in 2007 held at Harvard Medical School. This was followed up by international conferences in the Netherlands in 2009 and Vancouver, British Columbia, in 2012. Thousands of scientists and practitioners of all types—chiropractors, physical therapists, massage therapists, physicians, anybody interested in fascia—convened to share their theories, experience, and scientific research. Another congress is scheduled for Washington DC, in 2015, and the plan is to convene once every three years.

All of us physicians involved with fascia are learning things we never learned in medical school, because everything is new. It is quite exciting, but also confusing sometimes. For example, different researchers define fascia different ways, or classify fascia into various categories. For the purpose of the Fascial Distortion Model, fascia is seen as a collection of tissue that functions in interconnected layers. These layers then form a honeycomb-type structure.

Biotensegrity (Biological + Tension + Integrity)

Another great discovery is that fascia holds the human skeleton, muscles, and everything else together using a structural form known as *biotensegrity*. The core concept here is *tensegrity*, an idea developed by architect and inventor R. Buckminster Fuller. The word is a combination of *tension* and *integrity*, meaning that a structural whole is achieved (integrity) by using flexible components that exert tension on the rigid parts. Examples can be made with models using little sticks and rubber bands, or on a larger scale, the geodesic domes that Fuller developed. An even

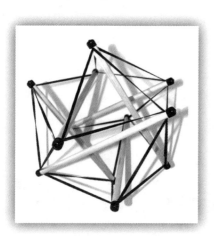

larger example is the Golden Gate Bridge, which is suspended with large cables that allow the rigid part of the bridge to be supported. In our medical model, when we look at your bone, muscle, or ligament from a distance, it is like seeing the span of the bridge. But as you get closer you can see the important role of the little cables of fascia that connect to that span. If you went and cut all of those cables, the bridge span would collapse into the water.

Beautiful sculptures, such as those in Vancouver's parks, visually explain the tensegrity model. Solid objects can be supported by thin flexible objects. The support of these solid structures in three-dimensional space is due to the tension inherent in the structure itself. The tension contained within the system is responsible for the integrity of the system.

*Bio*tensegrity is tensegrity applied to the biologic realm. The fibers in fascia exert tension on the bones, muscles, and ligaments that they attach to, and their flexibility allows the muscles to move the bones. The rigid bones are not directly connected to each other; they are held in place as an integrated system by the tensional pull of fascia. If we think of fascia as just a sheath or bandage, we are missing its true function. Then we're not getting the whole idea of the fascia as forming a matrix that allows a stabilized structure capable of fluent motion—the notion of biotensegrity. Dr. Donald Ingber and others have worked to explain biological systems down to the cellular level in terms of this principle.[7]

Sliding and Gliding

A French hand surgeon, Dr. J.C. Guimberteau, used a miniature camera to videotape fascia in action under the skin—in all its glorious biotensegrity. The movie shows the strings of fascia stretching and contracting and even changing form, meeting every request to morph and change structurally, an ability that offers infinite potential for mobility. The wispy strands appear delicate, but they are primarily composed of collagen with an amazingly high tensile strength. Don't be fooled; fascia is quite a challenge to deal with for the practitioner—and the source of a lot of tenacious pain for patients.

The video shows how layers of fascia serve as a kind of living lubricant, constantly adjusting to allow muscles and ligaments and bones to slide and glide past each other without any friction. During motion, the fibrous strands within the fascial layer extend and contract, making fluent activity possible.

If you cut a muscle in half, each little fiber within that muscle is wrapped with fascia, and each little bundle of muscle fibers is wrapped, and each bigger muscle group also has a wrapping. And between the muscle group and the skin is another layer of fascia called superficial fascia. It behaves as four or five layers that slide and glide on each other. But even within the muscles, they need to be moving and sliding. This freedom of fascial movement indicates a healthy system.

Distorted Fascia Causes Pain and Dysfunction

The opposite is also true. If the fascia is distorted, or somehow gets twisted, wrinkled, or torn, then movement is hindered and the person feels pain. The Fascial Distortion Model holds the position that fascia serves as a major pain receptor for the body (nociceptor), so in many cases the main source of pain from an injury is distorted fascia. And because fascia is wrapped around every cell in our bodies, any injury is liable to distort fascia. Therefore, the FDM manipulations can reduce pain in almost any injury.

It is generally accepted that acute pain is telling us something is wrong and we need to pay attention to it. For example, if your finger touches a hot stove, the heat activates a pain receptor that signals your autonomic nervous system to move it off the stove. But chronic pain is more mysterious. When an injury has apparently healed, there is no danger and therefore the ongoing pain seems to be sending a useless message. But looking at chronic pain through the FDM lens, often times there is still a valid message that something is wrong, and what is wrong is that the fascia is distorted. It makes sense that, if the pain receptor itself is all bunched up or torn, it's quite likely to send pain signals. That approach solved the pain in my elbows, and it solved the pain for my patient with the lacerated shin who limped around for two years. Both cases were treated by correcting the distortion through manipulation, thereby getting rid of the pain and restoring free movement.

With the understanding that distorted fascia alone can cause pain and limit movement, it becomes clear that some injuries are *only* distorted fascia and nothing more. This is true for many instances of pulled muscles and sprains. Conventional medicine holds that sprained ankles typically take weeks to heal, but FDM treatments can often fix them in a few minutes.

Saving the Game . . . for the Wrong Team

At a recent high school basketball game, a player from the visiting team sprained his ankle during the first half.

At halftime, he went to a local clinic and happened to get a physician who uses the Fascial Distortion Model. The physician used the medically accepted Ottawa rules to determine whether x-rays were warranted, and they were not. The injured player's description of the pain and his body language gave the physician enough clues to figure out what kind of a fascial distortion the boy had. The physician treated it very quickly, and the player was able to return to the game and play as if nothing had happened. In fact, his team won the game. If he had gone to any other kind of physician he would have walked out with crutches, ice, and painkillers, and would not have played for another couple of weeks. The physician who treated him, however, had mixed feelings. "I'm glad he was able to play right away, but because of it our team lost," he said. "Maybe I should have waited to treat him until after the game!"

The Dance Must Go On

FDM treatments can also provide significant pain relief when there is actual damage to the bone. After all, bones have no nerves, so why does it hurt when you break your arm? Because it's the distorted fascia surrounding the break that hurts, not the bone itself. That's why we can treat fractures and reduce the fascia pain. We cannot fix the fracture, but you can get pain relief.

I recently treated a sixteen-year-old ballet dancer with a stress fracture in her right shin. She was unable to walk up and down stairs using the affected leg other than as a support. She was unable to apply weight to the leg, and she could not push off. Ballet-style jumping was very painful in the area of the stress fracture. She initially went to an orthopedist who verified her stress fracture with x-rays. He treated her with ice, steroid medications, and a bone stimulator, but after a year the pain continued. The only thing she didn't do was take a prolonged rest.

When she came to see me, I examined and treated the area of the damaged shin. I found several small continuum distortions and a large triggerband. Correction of these seemed to cause significant immediate relief of her discomfort and pain.

I then asked her to demonstrate the ballet moves that gave her the most difficulty, and noticed her right calf was extremely stiff, which made her unable to do the move properly. She suspected that the tight calf muscle may have helped cause her stress fracture in the first place because it limited proper movement. I treated the calf and her Achilles tendon with multiple triggerband techniques. These treatments provided significant relief. She was able to climb the stairs with minimal pain, and after her third treatment, had no pain at all on the stairs.

She was also able to resume performing ballet jumps, but decided only to do them during rehearsals and performances and not during classes. I referred her back to an orthopedist for continued evaluations and x-rays. The stress fracture remained stable, and her pain kept decreasing. She was able to attend a seven-week intensive ballet camp on the East Coast with minimal discomfort even though the stress fracture continued. After one year of FDM treatments she felt no pain at all during her jumps, for the first time in two years.

The young dancer's tight calf muscle brings up a general point about fascia. Healthy fascia allows fluent motion, but the lack of sufficient motion and stretching allows the fascia to stiffen up. This underscores the constant need to stay active in order to keep your fascia supple and flexible. Lack of exercise, poor posture, or too much sitting at a desk can have ill effects that need to be corrected. Stiff fascia is unable to heal itself.

Stiff or frozen-tight fascia can also pull joints or body structures out of alignment. If we look at the problem through the lens of the biotensegrity model, we can see that the long-term solution is not to manipulate the joint by adjusting the bones. That's because the distorted fascia will just pull them out of whack again with their stubborn tensile strength. A patient might have some immediate relief, but it won't last. A more effective way to achieve symmetry and return the joint to a proper range of movement is to manipulate the fascia, the cause of the misalignment in the first place.

Fascia Facts

- Our body is truly an interconnected system.

- Fascia allows the body to move and function as a cohesive unit.

- Dysfunction of the fascia causes pain.

- Fascial distortions can have impact in the body at distant locations.

- Patients describe that pain in consistent fashion.

The Functions of Fascia

As the world of science advances, fascia is now thought to play a variety of important roles in many of our bodily processes:

Sensory

- Mechanoreceptor—a specialized sensory end organ that responds to mechanical stimuli such as tension, pressure, or displacement.

- Interoception—sensitive to stimuli outside the body

- Nociception—a source of pain sensations/pain receptors

Proprioceptive

- Unconscious perception of the body's orientation in space and movement, kind of an inner feedback mechanism

Supportive

- Biotensegrity—fascia applies tension to bones to create a flexible structure capable of movement.

Conductive

- Muscular force transmission—fascia helps the muscles exert force on the bones; muscles don't act alone

Contractile

- Fascia has the ability to contract. Previously it was thought that only muscle had this property. The fascia contractility is believed to play a role in the development of the body's tensegrity.

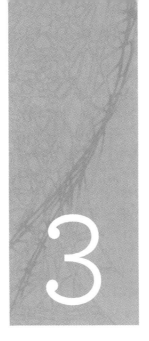

The Fascial Distortion Model: The Six Distortions

What Is a Model?

You can think of a model as a mental map or a mindset that guides providers when diagnosing and treating patients with musculoskeletal pain and injuries. Like a map, the model tells us what to look for and what to do when we find it. Dr. Stephen Typaldos was the creator of the Fascial Distortion Model, so he created the first map based on his assumptions, theories, and experience of what worked best for treating patients. The key topographical features on his map are the six basic kinds of distortions of fascia that he encountered, which will be described below.

The FDM visualizes the fascia in terms of its relationship to the entire body, with special consideration to the functional role it plays in movement. You might say we have an animated map that helps us visualize how the fascia functions during movement, and how it might be distorted when movement is limited and when the patient reports pain. In the medical profession, the model you are using guides your diagnosis, and the diagnosis directs the treatment.

The model is important to practitioners because we can't see the fascia, so we have to visualize it. For example, look at my dilemma in getting treatment for my tennis elbow from the conventional orthopedic model. The orthopedists couldn't see my fascia problem because it wasn't on their map. All they had was "inflammation." They "knew" that inflammation was the cause of my pain even if imaging failed to show any inflammation, and even if the treatment provided no relief for two years. They "knew" because their model told them so, even if it ran in the face of common sense. It's like the people who blame their faulty GPS systems for accidentally driving into a lake. Sometimes you have to say, "This model isn't working. It's time to try another model that does." For my tennis elbow, the new model was the FDM.

The Patient Is the Expert

The first basic assumption of the Fascial Distortion Model is that the patient intuitively knows what is wrong, and will show and tell the medical provider. After all, that is how Dr. Typaldos discovered distorted fascia in the first place: his patient told him what to do. That became his routine with subsequent patients, and now it is a crucial part of the model. As he treated more and more patients, he noticed patterns that associated the same types of verbal reports and body language with specific fascial distortions. These patterns also became part of the model, so that when we see them, they guide us toward the problem and the solution.

The FDM is therefore a partnership in which the provider must steadfastly listen to the patients and pay attention to their gestures. The discovery of fascial distortions would never have happened under the old model of the doctor/patient relationship, in which the physician did all the talking and the patient kept quiet. That was not a partnership; it was more of a one-sided activity, which unfortunately still happens all too often.

We believe the system of knowing and communicating pain in the fascia is inherent and therefore universal.[8] Patients intuitively know what needs to happen to feel better. People from all over the world communicate their pain in strikingly similar ways. This universal verbal and body language is what the FDM is based upon. As FDM providers, we learn to recognize this universal language of gestures, which allows us to make diagnoses of fascial distortions. We also rely on the patient to verify whether the pain is reduced after treatment. Without this information and feedback, we'd be flying blind. In the FDM, the patient is the expert.

The Fascial Distortion Model

The main topographical features of the "map" developed by Dr. Typaldos are the six primary distortions. Here is Dr. Typaldos' textbook definition of the Fascial Distortion Model:

"The fascial distortion model is an anatomical perspective in which most musculoskeletal injuries and certain medical conditions are envisioned as consisting of one or more of six principal fascial distortion types—each of which have signature clinical presentations." [9]

Triggerband: Distorted banded fascial tissue **(TB)**

Herniated Triggerpoint: Abnormal protrusion of tissue through fascial plane **(HTP)**

Continuum Distortion: Alteration of transition zone between ligament, tendon, other connective tissue, and bone **(CD)**

Folding Distortion: Three dimensional alteration of fascial plane **(FD)**

Cylinder Distortion: Overlapping of cylindrical fascial coils **(CyD)**

Tectonic Fixation: Alteration in ability of fascial surfaces to glide **(TF)**

These various distortions, which are often in combination, account for a wide variety of injuries and ailments that can be effectively treated through manipulation. In my experience, the first three are the most common. The primary tool for manipulation is the thumb, for although fascial distortions cannot be seen, most of them can be felt. In medical terminology, we say that the distorted fascia is *palpable*. Treatment is directed to the specific distortions, and once you treat them, they are gone. The anatomical injury no longer exists, and the patient can resume normal function, free of pain. This allows for some strikingly effective results, often for things that are typically really hard to treat, such as sprains, fractures, frozen shoulders, and other soft tissue injuries. The FDM is also effective in the treatment of other musculoskeletal and neurologic conditions that previously had limited treatment options. Treatment of these fascial distortions allows the fascial matrix to regain its normal function. When the fascia is free once again to move in its normal function of sliding and gliding with the rest of the body, the pain melts away.

1. Triggerband (TB)

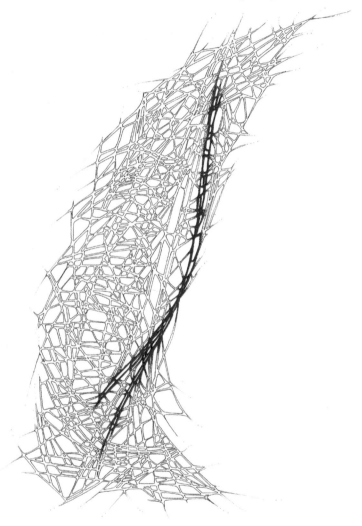

A **triggerband** is distorted banded fascial tissue. This is a relatively common type of fascial distortion and the easiest to repair. It was the first distortion to be identified by Dr. Typaldos.

Subjective Description

Patients say they feel a line of pain along with a pulling or burning sensation. They may describe a weakness of the limb in certain positions, and say it feels tight. Patients may also report a loss of balance.

Body Language

Patients indicate the pain with a sweeping motion using one or more fingers, usually showing the pain going along a line.

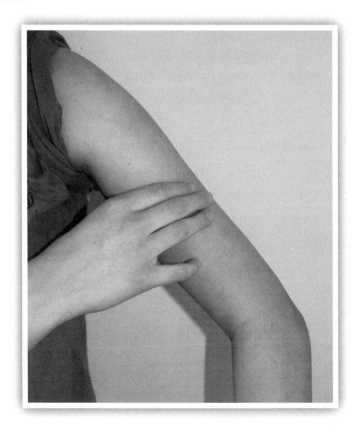

FDM Analysis/Observation

Although we envision the fascia as a matrix throughout the body, sometimes it appears to function in part as bands or linear sheets. Like a sheet, the band of fascia can become torn, wrinkled, or twisted. This is what causes the pain and inhibits movement.

Triggerbands can start suddenly as in an acute injury. The abnormal tension of the initial triggerband may cause secondary triggerbands to form over time. These triggerbands may last for a long time until they are treated, and they can develop adhesions to other structures. Triggerbands can be associated with other distortions, including herniated triggerpoints (HTPs), continuum distortions (CDs), and cylinder distortions (CyDs).

There is often a loss of range of movement (ROM) in one or more planes of motion related to a joint.

How It Feels to the Practitioner

Triggerbands often feel like a ribbon or string going along the band, often about the size of a violin string.

Treatment

You can correct a triggerband by applying force with the thumb to essentially iron out the twist or wrinkle. Untwisting the fascial fibers gets them back in proper position to reattach, somewhat like closing a resealable plastic bag. When a resealable plastic bag is opened, the ends of the zipper portion become closer together. This is analogous to the pulling and tightness patients feel and consistently describe. As the bag is closed, the ends separate, thereby relieving the tension within the system and providing pain relief.

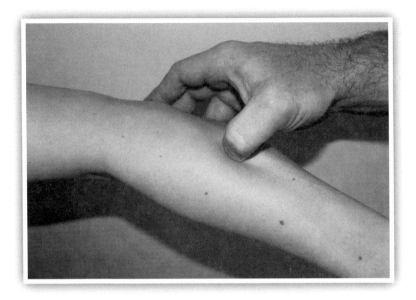

The pain starts and stops at an end point. Pain or pressure is identified along the entire pathway.

The patient can speed recovery by moving the affected part. No matter how tired my patients feel after a treatment, I advise them to go for a walk right away or the next day, and to walk thirty to sixty minutes every day. Fascia is designed to move, and activity is the best prescription.

Warning

I strongly advise against applying heat; electrical stimulation; and rest. Heat feels good at the time, but the pain comes back strongly as soon as it is removed. My theory is that heat bakes the layers of fascia together, decreasing the fascia's ability to move and providing temporary relief. Once the heat effect wears off the fascia is free to move, and the fascial pain returns—sometimes with even greater intensity. The same goes for electrical stimulation. Rest also allows the fascia to stiffen into place, essentially stalling the healing process and making the problem worse.

Possible Outcomes

A triggerband can have several possible outcomes once it has developed in the body.

1. You can repair it immediately with FDM treatment.

2. The body can heal it slowly on its own.

3. The triggerband may persist in its initial state without developing adhesions to surrounding tissues.

4. The triggerband may become stuck to other tissues and become chronic.

Quick Guide to Triggerband Distortions

- **Symptoms**: Burning, pulling, pain along a line

- **Body Language**: Sweeping motion with fingers along painful linear pathway

- **Problem**: Twisted or wrinkled band of fascia

- **Feels Like**: A ribbon or violin string

- **Treatment**: Use thumb to untwist and iron out the wrinkled tissue.

- **Warning**: Stay away from heat and electrical stimulation; don't rest.

2. Herniated Triggerpoint (HTP)

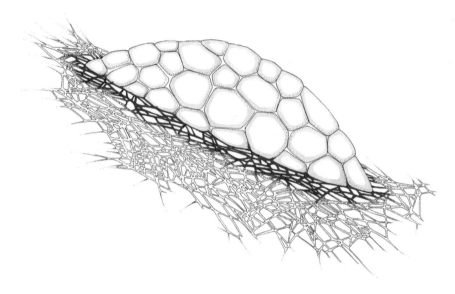

A herniated triggerpoint is an abnormal protrusion of tissue through a fascial plane. I see more patients with HTPs than any other distortion.

Subjective Description

Patients describe the pain associated with this distortion as an ache, pinching, or catching.

Body Language

Patients indicate the ache by pressing or pushing their thumb or multiple fingers into the tender protruding tissue. (Patients will sometimes admit to having a spouse or friend press on these areas. Some patients will try to use a ball or other physical tool to press them back in place.)

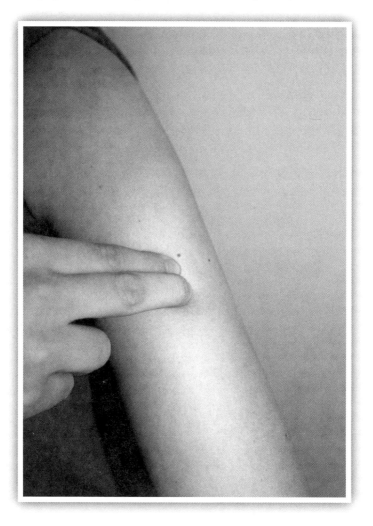

FDM Analysis/Observation

This distortion is also based on the theory that the fascial matrix sometimes functions as a sheet or a layer. One or more layers of fascial tissue can have another tissue protrude through them, restricting free motion. HTPs may occur suddenly though a trauma associated with a slip and fall, or when bending over to pick something up. They also may develop from no apparent cause over time. Often patients say they just woke up one day with the deep ache.

HTPs are considered to be permanent unless they are treated; they don't go away by themselves. They may fluctuate in intensity, but until the tissue is pushed back through the layer that has been penetrated, they will not go away. HTPs often result in the decreased ROM of contiguous joints. There can be a "stepping" or hesitant motion of the joint nearest the HTP.

Some HTPs may be associated with triggerbands. So-called banded HTPs may be quite large. A fascial tear may allow for a significant amount of tissue to press through a layer of fascia. Some of these are so large I envision them as a fascial rent, a large tear that allows fat, fascia, or other soft tissue to protrude through.

How It Feels to the Practitioner

Often there is a palpable knot of soft tissue in the area of pain.

Treatment

The practitioner uses the thumb to push the protruding tissue back below the fascial plane. Proper direction of force is important for achieving reduction. Treatment of HTPs can be quite painful and may sometimes result in a significant bruise.

Patients can get relief and improved ROM when the HTP is pressed. The relief will be temporary, however, unless the protruding tissue is completely pushed back beneath the fascial layer.

Comment

I see the same places for herniated triggerpoints over and over again. Here are some of the common locations for HTPs:

- Supraclavicular—on top of the collarbone

- Bull's-eye—in the butt cheek

- Abdomen

- Flank—the side between the last rib and the hip

- Lumbar—on the back between the bottom rib and the pelvis

- Deltoid—thick triangular muscle covering the shoulder joint

- Subscapularis—on the outside edge of the scapula below the shoulder in the back

- Subacromial—at the point of the shoulder

Coincidence or Connection?

In an effort to explain why some areas in the body are so susceptible to HTPs, my partner (an osteopathic physician) and I researched anatomy books. We found a correlation between frequent HTP spots and the location of superficial subcutaneous nerves. Is there a connection?

Quick Guide to Herniated Triggerpoints

- **Symptoms**: An ache, pinching, or catching

- **Body Language**: Pushes the thumb or fingers into a specific spot

- **Problem**: Tissue is protruding through a rupture in a layer of fascia.

- **Feels Like**: a knot or a grape

- **Treatment**: Push the knot back through the hole in the fascia.

- **Warning**: HTPs are permanent unless treated.

3. Continuum Distortion (CD)

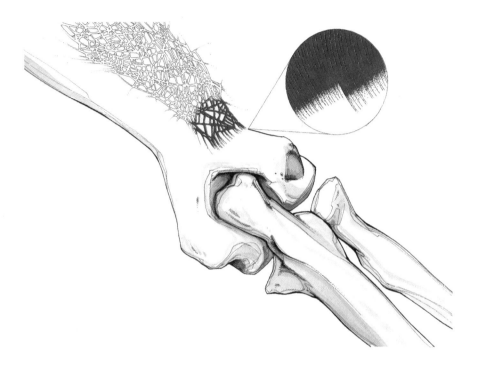

A continuum distortion is an alteration of the transition zone between ligament, tendon, and other connective tissue and bone.

Subjective Description

The patient will complain of pain on one spot on a bone. There may be multiple CDs in an area but they are all described as individual spots of pain.

Body Language

The pain is identified with a single finger pointing to one specific spot, usually near a joint line where the fascia covering a ligament, tendon, or muscle inserts into the periosteum of the bone.

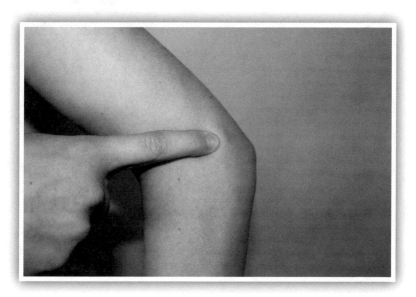

FDM Analysis/Observation

The connection between fascia and the bone is not a static one because the fascia keeps rapidly changing between being flexible and being rigid, depending on the needs of any particular action. This is part of its biotensegrity function. The place where fascia and bone meet is a transition zone, or continuum, that involves the flow of calcium molecules back and forth between the bone and the fascia. When the fascia needs to be rigid, calcium flows into it; when it needs to be flexible, the calcium flows back to the bone. If this transitioning is interrupted by some unexpected action, such as twisting your ankle on a basketball court, then the transition is suspended halfway between being rigid and being flexible. The result is intense pain and limited movement, such as being unable to walk on a sprained ankle.

How It Feels to the Practitioner

A continuum distortion often feels like a tiny grain of rice, or a pen tip.

Treatment

The practitioner applies force with the thumb to cause the transition zone to shift. When the shift occurs, it feels like a pimple popping or butter melting.

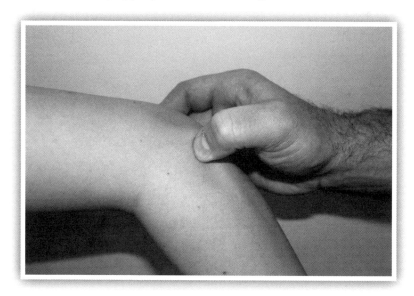

Progression of a Continuum Distortion

- The CD occurs suddenly.

- It could last a long time, or shift back to normal on its own.

- It may come and go with activity.

- CDs may cause triggerbands.

- Often CDs cause loss of flexion/extension in a joint.

Quick Guide to Continuum Distortions

- **Symptoms**: A specific spot of pain on a bone.

- **Body Language**: Single finger points to a specific spot

- **Problem**: Sudden movement disrupts the fascia's fluid connection to the bone.

- **Feels Like**: A small grain of rice

- **Treatment**: Push on the distortion until it shifts, pops, or melts, thus shifting back to neutral.

4. Folding Distortion (FD)

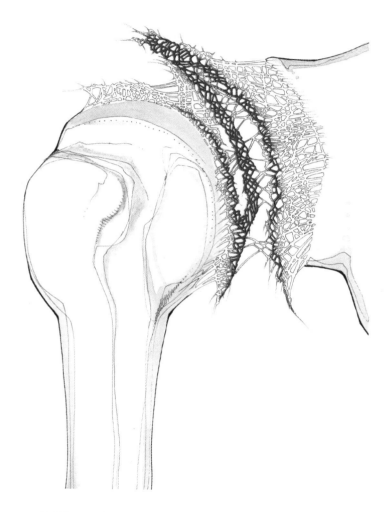

A folding distortion is a three-dimensional alteration of a fascial plane. It is most often found in a joint, such as the wrist, elbow, or shoulder. It can also occur in the areas between muscles and between bones.

Subjective Description

Patients will describe the pain in a joint as "deep in there somewhere." They will report a painful range of movement, but usually there is no significant loss of motion. Since these distortions can remain unchanged over a long period of time, they will describe it as their "usual pain" or the "pain I've always had." They sometimes say the joint feels unstable.

Body Language

Patients cup the joint with the palm of their hands, or they will squeeze the joint.

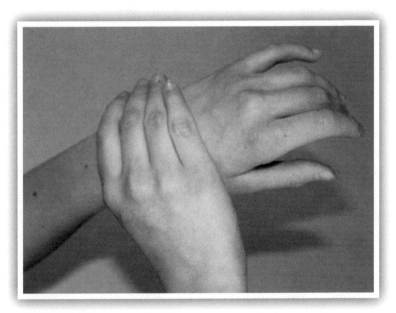

If the folding distortion is between muscles or between bones, patients will press fingers deep into the gap between the two.

FDM Analysis/Observation

Folding distortions occur most often in hinge joints where the fascia needs to open and close like an accordion. The distortion occurs when the fascia gets stuck unfolding open or stuck while refolding shut. The story is that Dr. Typaldos was at a theater and got the idea when he saw the curtains open and close like an accordion. Another classic analogy to illustrate FDs is the folding of a road map. If you unfold the road map all the way and twist it slightly, the map gets stuck and can't close. The same thing occurs if the map is compressed and distorted while refolding, because then the map will not be able to fully reopen. Injuries involving refolding and unfolding are fairly common.

Examples of unfolding injuries are when a joint is stretched out, such as in bungee jumping, when a parachute opens during a jump, or when a dog pulls suddenly on a leash. The joint fascia is unfolded open and can't close. Examples of refolding injuries are when you jam your wrist when falling down with an open hand, or when your finger is jammed with a basketball. The joint fascia is compressed and can't reopen. Such injuries can be permanent unless they are treated; they do not heal themselves. Sometimes the joint swells if the body is trying to unfold the fascia.

While foldings are most commonly thought of as being in a joint, the fascia between muscles or between bones can also distort in a refolding and unfolding manner.

How It Feels to the Practitioner

You cannot feel the FD because it is inside a joint, between muscles, or between bones.

Treatment

Treatment of these distortions involves recreating the initial injury. The positive side to fixing these distortions is that the direction of treatment is the direction that doesn't cause pain. So a refolding injury feels better when compressed. Therefore, the joint is treated with a compression thrust technique. For example, you treat a jammed finger by pushing it in, and when it gets back into place, you'll hear a pop.

Unfolding injuries feel better with traction (pulling). Traction thrust techniques are applied to correct unfolding injuries. When successfully treating an unfolding, you will often hear a click while pulling it into place. If a folding distortion is being treated and pain is present, then either the diagnosis is incorrect or other distortions are present that should be addressed before the folding distortion is treated.

Progression of a Folding Distortion

- The FD occurs suddenly as a trauma.

- It remains unchanged until re/unfolded.

- It's considered permanent until corrected.

Quick Guide to Folding Distortions

- **Symptoms**: Deep ache in the joint that feels like it restricts movement, but when tested, the range of motion is normal.

- **Body Language**: Patient cups hands over the joint

- **Problem**: Accordion-like fascia gets stuck after opening or closing too far.

- **Treatment**: Repeat the injury: pull on an unfolding and push on a refolding.

- **Good News**: This treatment is not painful.

- **Bad News**: Distortion is permanent unless treated.

5. Cylinder Distortion (CyD)

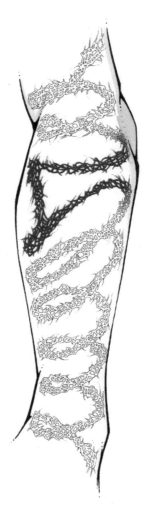

A cylinder distortion is the overlapping of cylindrical fascial coils. This is the most bizarre, mysterious, and elusive distortion. Providers not using the FDM may suspect the problem is merely psychological.

Subjective Description

Patients with a CyD will describe a seemingly bizarre pain that is very difficult to pinpoint and may actually jump from place to place on the body. The patient may also report a variety of uncomfortable sensations including numbness, tingling, "pins and needles" (paresthesia), a feeling of swelling when there is no swelling, and even tremor. Patients will often verbally struggle to explain the pain, saying, "It depends." Pain may come at night in the form of cramping. The pain can be felt deep in the body, but sometimes a light touch can cause pain of inexplicable intensity.

Body Language

The patient repeatedly squeezes and sweeps the palm over the area of pain. Sometimes it appears that he or she is trying to sweep the pain away or trying to remove a glove or sock.

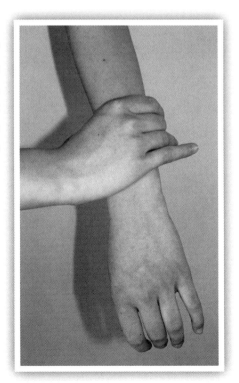

FDM Analysis/Observation

The mysterious pain with no apparent anatomical cause is due to tangled cylindrical fascia that encompasses the surface of the body under the skin. Imagine the body coated in a spiral netting of coils, somewhat like a Slinky toy. When these coils of fascia get tangled, a patient can feel pain as well as a variety of other sensations. Generally cylinder distortions occur over the non-jointed portions of the body in the trunk and extremities. We cannot see literal coils of fascia, but rather that is how we visualize its presumed function in this distortion.

Cylinder distortions often start suddenly without apparent cause. They can also be the result of having to wear splints, casts, taping, or other kinds of immobilization. Cylinder distortions can also be caused by tight clothing or other fascial distortions such as triggerbands.

Patients with cylinder distortions can have pain with active motion but can be pain-free in passive motion. The pain of cylinder distortions is often out of proportion to physical findings. Sometimes swelling (edema) may be associated with cylinder distortions.

How It Feels to the Practitioner

The area where a cylinder distortion is located may feel normal, so sometimes a pet comb can be used to identify the tangled coils just under the skin. Once the tangle is identified, patients and practitioners will often be able to feel them.

Treatment

Treatment of cylinder distortions is directed at trying to untangle the coiled fascia. Different techniques using the hands can be applied. Many massage techniques may actually be treating the cylinder fascia. Other tools such as cups, clips, and clamps may be utilized to try and uncoil the fascia. I have even used a vacuum device designed for assisting in childbirth. Sometimes cylinder distortions can actually be caused by some of the treatment techniques in the FDM. So it's important to remember that it is possible to overdo the treatment and cause more cylinders. Treatment of the cylinder can induce dramatic reduction of visible swelling.

Warning

Between the bizarre descriptions of pain and the lack of apparent physical cause, a conventional physician may question the reality of the pain and refer the patient to a psychiatrist.

Possible Outcomes

The progression of a cylinder distortion is unpredictable.

Quick Guide to Cylinder Distortions

- **Symptoms**: bizarre symptoms such as pain that fluctuates or jumps from one area to another, numbness, tingling, tremor, impression of swelling

- **Body Language**: Hand appears to squeeze or sweep the pain away.

- **Problem**: Coiled fascia under the skin gets tangled.

- **Feels Like**: Difficult to feel; may have to use a pet comb to find tangle

- **Treatment**: Untangle fascia coils with hands, cups, pet comb, baby-vac, and so on.

- **Warning**: Conventional physician may refer patient to a psychiatrist.

6. Tectonic Fixation (TF)

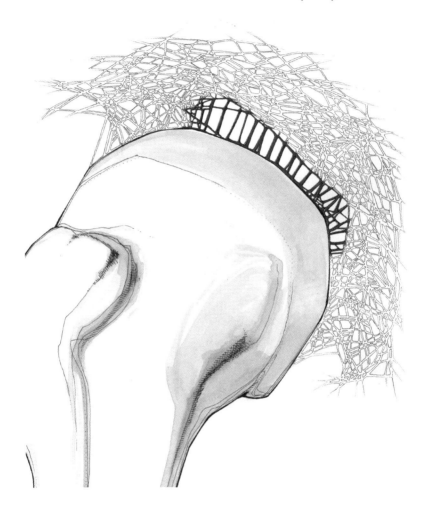

A tectonic fixation is an inability of the fascial surfaces to glide, so they are stuck together. A frozen shoulder is a common example.

Subjective Description

Patients will say that a shoulder feels: "stiff," "like it needs to pop," "stuck," or "like I am a quart low on oil."

Body Language

Patient has stiff joint movement and tries to move joint with force. Patient may grab one part of the joint and jiggle it to try to get relief.

FDM Analysis/Observation

Tectonic fixations occur when the fascial matrix has lost the ability of its surfaces to glide. The surfaces of the fascial layers are attracted to one another—as if by magnetic pull—and motion is not possible.

Tectonic fixations often begin slowly. This distortion is often a ramification of the pain and immobilization caused by other distortions. The progression of a tectonic fixation is dependent on its underlying cause.

A tectonic fixation has a decreased ROM when moved. The joint involved has severe restriction in motion. Often the restriction or end point feels distinct and boney, almost as if the restriction in the joint has formed due to bones striking one another. Tectonic fixations do not hurt when they are palpated.

How It Feels to the Practitioner

The TF is not palpable because it is inside a joint. Decreased ROM is evident when a joint is tested.

Treatment

Techniques used to treat tectonic fixations may include manipulation in the form of slowly pumping joint fluid between the layers of fascia, followed by joint mobilization. The goal is to restore the fascial surface's ability to glide. This is the only distortion for which heat may be beneficial. Before treatment, heat and gentle stretching will increase the fluidity of the joint lubricant.

Quick Guide to Tectonic Fixations

- **Symptoms**: Joint that won't move.

- **Body Language**: Grabs joint and tries to jiggle it; tries to move joint with force.

- **Problem**: The fascial layers are stuck to each other instead of gliding.

- **Treatment**: Slow pumping of fluid between the layers, followed by joint mobilization; heat may increase fluidity of the joint lubricant.

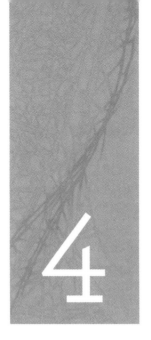

The Model Applied:
Common Conditions

The Fascial Distortion Model has proven its value to me and my patients for its effectiveness in reducing pain and restoring freedom of movement. There is nothing more rewarding to a physician than to successfully treat somebody who had been frustrated with other forms of treatment, and perhaps suffered for years. I am frequently humbled by their thankfulness in finding relief. As a result, I now devote my practice entirely to manipulation, both FDM techniques and the osteopathic manipulations I learned in medical school. I am continually astonished—as are my patients—by the profound relief that comes from such a simple treatment.

I have found that the key to success is to stick with the model, listen to the patients, and let their descriptions and body language be my guide. I am getting better at reading their body language, and sometimes I am tempted to jump the gun and prematurely arrive at a diagnosis. This is a mistake, because patients often have problems that involve more than one distortion. I'm constantly reminding myself to stick with the model. That is also my mantra when training other physicians to use the FDM: "Stick with the model!"

The FDM manipulations work with all kinds of musculoskeletal injuries, but in the next two chapters, I'll examine some of the common problems that I help my patients face. Therefore, I will not present a comprehensive list of the range of problems that can be treated, but rather just a sampling of case histories to give an idea of how effective the model can be when applied to actual cases.

Back Pain

Back pain is one of the most common reasons I see patients. I have found that back pain means something different to nearly everyone. When patients complain of back pain and I ask them to show me where it hurts, some will point to the base of the neck, others indicate the lower back, and some will point to the buttock. So the complaint of back pain is actually pretty vague. Needless to say, many different distortions are responsible for this array of different pains—all lumped together as "back pain."

Standing Tall

One patient in her sixties with a diagnosis of fibromyalgia came to me complaining of back pain. The first time I saw her she walked in bent over at the waist at a forty-five-degree angle, and was using a cane for support. Apparently she had not stood up straight for many years.

Her pain was in the low back and she described a band-like pain running up and down either side of the spine. She also pressed with multiple fingers into several sore areas in the low back. Despite her bent-over posture, she was able to live in her cabin outside of the city, which included heating her home with wood. I treated her for herniated trigger-points and triggerband distortions, which enabled her to stand up straight.

She was thrilled to be able to straighten up for the first time in years. As with all my patients, I encouraged her to walk. I wanted her to get out and be active so the fascial tissue could get moving. That day she felt quite good—better than she had in years—so she left my office and decided to walk home. She made it three miles before she got tired and had to call for a ride. At our next visit, she laughed about this impulsive choice. She forgot to think about getting tired from a heart and lung perspective. Her back pain had been so severe, it had been years since she was able to perform any type of exercise to keep her heart and lungs in good condition.

Paratrooper

Living in Alaska, I have the pleasure of working with some of the military personnel stationed in our communities. Military physicians have learned of the possible benefits of the Fascial Distortion Model for the soldiers and their families, so they frequently refer patients to my partners and me. I have performed FDM treatments on many of these soldiers with good results, enabling them to return to full duty. The soldiers started calling me the "Back Ninja."

One soldier was a paratrooper before coming to Alaska. Unfortunately, his parachuting ended on a bad jump when his chute got caught on a tree. As he fell toward the ground, he got tangled up in the lines until he was hanging upside down. Apparently, he was suspended there as if on a spring, and bounced up and down, striking his helmeted head on the ground until he passed out. When he woke up, he had to cut the ropes to free himself. He developed both upper and lower back pain, as well as a numbness and tingling in his heel. He had extensive treatment and imaging. He underwent numerous MRI exams, prolonged physical therapy, and saw pain physicians who had performed numerous injections and radio-ablative procedures in an effort to get his pain under control. He also took a fairly large amount of narcotic medications. He saw a neurologist and had an MRI. Nothing relieved the back pain or numbness in his heel for any length of time.

By the time he finally came to me, it was years after his injury. I soon discovered he had virtually all types of distortions in his back and on his body. As I treated him we worked through a lot of those issues. He found the first treatment to be intensely painful. Afterward he felt like he was moving better and was in less pain, and that allowed him to sleep better. Still—as I found out later—he was unsure of the true value of that treatment because he was looking for some definitive sign that he was doing better.

On the second treatment, I found a herniated trigger-point between two ribs just below his right shoulder blade. As soon as I reduced the HTP, he immediately noticed that the numbness in his heel vanished. We were both thrilled to see that chronic problem resolved. It was at that point that he became a believer in the FDM.

I worked with him on a monthly basis for about a year. During one of the visits about nine months into our treatments, he told me the numbness in his heel had started to come back. I immediately thought that the return of numbness was related to the spinal nerves in his low back. But then he reminded me that we had been able to correct the dead feeling by treating the HTP in his ribs. Listening to the patient, I looked for and found the HTP in the spot he remembered from that second treatment. I was able to reduce the HTP with minimal effort and, almost immediately, he reported that the tingling and numbness in his heel was gone once again. I continued to see him on a monthly basis until he retired from the military, and the issue with the heel never returned. His back pain was significantly reduced and his use of narcotic medications was drastically cut back. He was able to be much more active in everyday life, and resumed running.

Bull's-eye Herniated Triggerpoint (HTP)

You may recall that the distortion known as a herniated triggerpoint is considered permanent until treated. This means that patients may endure immobilizing pain for months or years, when all they need is a brief FDM treatment to solve the problem.

A case in point is an HTP in the butt cheek, a malady we refer to as a "bull's-eye" HTP. One patient had been volunteering in Haiti and came to me with a bull's-eye. The pain was so bad that she said she had trouble sleeping, she could barely walk, and it was troubling to even move. It was so painful that she couldn't even cross her legs while sitting on the treatment table. She pointed to the pain with a single finger, which confirmed for me that she was suffering from an HTP.

It took me fifteen minutes to explain to her what I was going to do, and about thirty seconds to fix the issue. She stood up and said, "What was that?" She sat down and was able to cross her legs. "No way! And I've been dealing with this for a year?"

Yes, after a year with a pain in the butt cheek, she was returned to mobility in less than a minute.

Headaches

A lot of patients come to me with headaches. I had an older woman patient from a nursing home who complained about painful spots on her scalp. She had these for years and would push on them. Sometimes she even banged her head on the wall in an effort to get rid of them.

That behavior was not appreciated at the nursing home, and everyone kind of chalked her up as being old and somewhat senile. But she came to me and described the painful spots on her skull. According to the FDM, I classified them as continuum distortions. I explained to her that I was going to push on her head. She was so thrilled because it validated her natural impulse. The first thing I did was give her the ability to say, "This is where it hurts."

As I pushed on it, I could feel the subtle change, and she would say, "Okay, that is better. Now there is one over here." We did that for probably three or four treatments and her headaches were dramatically reduced. Now she no longer has to bang her head on the wall to raise the ire of the nursing home attendants.

The FDM can deal with a variety of headaches, because a lot of them are not intracranial but outside the skull. There is a common kind of headache that will often be called a tension headache, musculoskeletal headache, or cervicogenic headache—those that come from your neck or neck pain—addressing those issues with manipulation is definitely a possibility.

Chronic Rib Pain

Some cases are complex and mysterious; yet even then, Fascial Distortion Model techniques can have a positive though limited effect. One such case is a woman who had chronic rib pain that began nine years earlier following a severe gastrointestinal illness. She had been extremely ill and vomited profusely. Then she had developed pain on her front-left chest associated with a specific rib (left anterior T 10). Of course, that location immediately makes physicians wonder about the heart, not to mention intra-abdominal organs and the colon. The patient underwent an upper endoscopy and colonoscopy to evaluate the possible causes of her pain. She had a CT scan of her chest, as well as a CT myelogram of the spine to try to determine whether there had been some damage in her spine that could explain this pain on the left side of her body.

This had been going on for approximately *nine years*. The pain had been disabling at times, and she suffered severe spasms and cramping that had prevented her from engaging in normal activity. When she came to me, she described the pain as a "rolling of her rib" accompanied by severe spasms. She responded pretty well to triggerband and herniated triggerpoint distortion techniques, as well as continuum distortion techniques to the rib. These treatments reduced her symptoms. She continues to have episodes where the pain returns, though overall it appears to be less intense. I have referred her to a massage therapist who understands the FDM. This has helped identify a possible connection in the shoulder fascia that may be contributing to her restricted motion, which may be preventing a total recovery of the rib. The treatments decreased her symptoms but did not totally resolve the issue. She continues to struggle with the rib pain and we are working on a course of treatment involving multiple different medical specialists to try and find her relief. Unfortunately, addressing the shoulder has triggered another shoulder pain that wasn't there previously. Whether this is an adverse effect of the treatment or a previously unrecognized connection remains to be determined.

Her story is similar to those of other patients who respond favorably to treatment and show good improvement, yet become very frustrated when the symptoms return after a period of months. I am not able to provide these patients the answer to the question they always have, "Why do these distortions sometimes come back?" Sometimes the distortions are treated completely and relief is long lasting. In other cases, relief occurs but the pain returns. In these situations, the goal of manipulation should be to provide relief while searching for the underlying cause of the pain and distortions' return.

Pelvic Pain

Pelvic pain is very difficult to treat because it can be caused by a variety of factors. It is also difficult in the sense that patients are often embarrassed about describing pain in the pelvic region. However, I have had several patients come forward to discuss this problem because it can be very life altering.

One patient in her sixties had been seeing me for about six months to work on her back pain. We had made good progress on her symptoms, and she had been able to increase her activity. As she became more comfortable with me, she confided that she had a pain in her pelvic region that had been bothering her since she was thirteen years old. As I listened to her description and watched her body language, it became apparent to me that she was describing a fascial distortion associated with a herniated triggerpoint in her groin area (inguinal).

I obtained a chaperone nurse to accompany me and I treated the HTP, a true hernia of fascia instead of the more familiar type of hernia that can contain abdominal content. Once again, this is a type of fascial distortion considered to be permanent until treated. The successful reduction of this hernia allowed for immediate improvement of a highly personal pain that had been bothering the patient for nearly fifty years.

She returned several weeks later with tears in her eyes and said, "I never knew it was possible to live without that pain. Now you have to treat the other side."

I was able to treat the alternate side just as effectively, and this woman's many years of pelvic discomfort and pain were gone. A dramatic benefit was that she learned sexual activity could be performed without pain.

I have had several other patients with various pelvic complaints, often described as a pain deep in the groin or the edge of the buttock between the sacrum (a complex bone in the back of the pelvis) and the perineum (the area from the rectum to the urogenital passages). This pain is often extremely uncomfortable and limits the patient's activity.

The area of the pain makes it somewhat embarrassing for a patient to discuss the problem with health-care providers, much less describe it in any detail. When he or she does eventually identify this pain, often it's confided to an obstetrician or primary care physician.

There are entire specialties devoted to pelvic pain. I had the good fortune of working with an obstetrician who had completed a pelvic pain fellowship. While she was working at our clinic we did conjoined visits, where we would look at a patient's complaint of pelvic pain from both of our perspectives. She had the perspective of surgical intervention, though she was very hesitant to perform any surgery on pelvic pain, as she often saw that as an excessive treatment. She often preferred injection therapy as a more appropriate tool. Between the two of us combining our treatments on these cases, we had at least a 50 percent improvement on our patients overall. Even a slight improvement in a patient's pelvic pain is considered a small victory.

Abdominal Pain

One patient came to me after suffering for years from a chronic pain in her abdomen. It had developed some time after a surgery to repair an umbilical hernia. She was in pain every day, which prevented her from participating in activities with her family and enjoying many other aspects of her life.

She sought help throughout the health-care system over the years. She was given an upper and lower endoscopy in the form of an EGD and a colonoscopy. She had a CT of the abdomen several times, with and without contrast. She had extensive blood work performed. She had an ultrasound to see if she had another hernia. When her pain continued, she was convinced to undergo another colonoscopy. One provider suggested exploratory surgery, and she was considering this option when she came to me.

She pointed to several areas of pain just to the right of her belly button. She used several fingers to indicate these areas of pain. She pressed into these areas and explained an aching in the abdomen near her hernia surgery.

I recognized this as several herniated triggerpoints on her abdominal wall, and performed treatments to relieve her pain. The relief was instantaneous. She was without pain for the first time in years.

At times like this, I have to stop and wonder why patients like her have to needlessly suffer for years. I think of the many thousands of dollars spent in the health-care system that could have been saved if someone had been trained to recognize the problem as a fascial distortion rather than looking past it.

Mastectomy Complications: Chest Wall Pain

Fascia generally becomes distorted through accident or injury, but can also happen as a side effect of surgery. The most profoundly disrupted fascia I have seen in post-surgery is that of women who have had double mastectomies as the ultimate treatment for breast cancer. These patients suffer from chest wall pain and a severe tightness that prevents them from catching a full breath. Even though they have recovered from the cancer itself, the musculoskeletal concerns can linger for years, limiting their ability to resume normal active lives.

A series of simple FDM treatments can restore a patient's ability to embrace life following a double mastectomy. Some post-breast cancer patients have responded very well to treatment of the anterior chest wall fascia with a resolution of the band-like tightness that they describe.

Breast Cancer Patient #1

Although I have conditioned myself to listen to the patient, one woman with a double mastectomy let her adult daughter do most of the talking. She described how her mother's pain in the chest was so severe, she couldn't exercise and wasn't even able to walk for any length of time. I coaxed the patient, who appeared visibly depressed, into describing the banded pain across the surgical scars on the front of her chest. She said a line of pain was in the scar. It had been many years since her surgery, so she had been suffering for a long time. She had survived cancer, but the residual pain had greatly diminished the quality of her life. No wonder she seemed depressed.

It was easy for me to visualize that the surgery had damaged the fascia on her chest, so I treated her with triggerband technique and corrected several small herniated triggerpoints within the front of the chest wall. I also found and treated some cylinder distortions in the same area. The patient seemed relieved right away and, with renewed freedom to move her chest, was able to take deep breaths.

When they returned for another treatment two weeks later, I was happily surprised to find that, this time, the patient did most of the talking and the daughter only occasionally chimed in. The patient reported that the treatment had gone very well. She said the band had loosened around her chest, and she was able to increase her physical activity. Her sense of relief was obvious. She appeared visibly more animated with better color, and was less depressed.

A month later, for her third treatment, the patient showed up without her daughter. As we talked about her progress, I mentioned that she probably would not need further treatments. She was relieved to hear this, and even joked about the difficulty of getting an appointment with me.

I was determining how to move forward at that time in my practice and I mentioned to her that I would likely start doing a full-time manipulation practice. She was somewhat startled by this revelation and asked, "Is that what you really want to do?"

I was struck by the phrase "really want to do." She viewed me as a family practice physician at the walk-in clinic who was doing additional manipulation. Yet she lamented how difficult it was to obtain an appointment with me. I thought for a moment and said that because of stories like hers, I felt it was my obligation to commit to doing full-time osteo-pathic manipulation using the Fascial Distortion Model.

She was a little bit confused by my comment, and questioned the part about "stories like hers." She did not fully understand the change I saw in her over those three visits. She had come to me as a depressed shell of herself, someone who was unable to be physically active and engaged in life around her. With simple treatments that allowed the tissues in her chest to move freely, she was able to regain her sense of vitality.

When I told her that she had looked quite depressed during that first visit, she was a little bit startled at the revelation. She denied that she was depressed at all. I brought up the fact that she had her daughter do all of the talking for her on the first visit, and pointed out the progression in the next two visits. On the second visit her daughter was merely a chaperone, and on the third visit her daughter didn't show up at all. I could see the glimmer of recognition in my patient's eyes as she realized the truth of her depression and how important the musculoskeletal pain post-surgery had been for her. This change in her persona had been life-altering based on the few principles of the FDM and the power of correcting her distortions.

Breast Cancer Patient #2

A different patient with a double mastectomy had especially deep surgery because her cancer had been detected close to the bones on her chest. She told me that it felt like someone was tightening a hose clamp on her chest. Moving her upper body was very difficult, and it was terribly painful to raise her arms. She was also troubled by the thick and discolored scar tissue left from the surgery. It was all purple and red and did not look like skin at all.

The fascia was obviously severely damaged, and so much muscle had been removed by the surgery that her skin was virtually adhering onto her bone. I treated trigger-bands, herniated triggerpoints, continuum distortions, and cylinder distortions.

She reported that after one treatment, she couldn't believe how much better she felt. Her insurance company would allow her to be treated by me just once per month, but fortunately she found a physical therapist who could manipulate the fascia to prevent it from freezing up between treatments. This was important because the fascia needed to become flexible before the patient could begin to move her upper body freely.

After several treatments, her ability to move without pain increased remarkably. She knew she needed to keep the fascia moving, so she deliberately placed objects on high shelves around her house to force herself to use her arms and upper body more. She also started to lift weights, and recently went kayaking.

She told me, "I feel like I have my freedom back! I'm able to reach higher and I don't have the pain. I just feel more alive than I used to."

I have come to expect such amazing results regarding decreased pain and increased movement, but the big surprise to me was the improvement in her scar tissue from the FDM treatments. She had been considering surgery to reduce the scar tissue, but after the treatments, it went down by itself and its color improved. She said, "I feel better when I look in the mirror and don't see purple and red, and my scar tissue is lying down more." The reduction was so significant that her prosthetics no longer fit. Her surgeon was also stunned by the change in her scar tissue when she saw him for a follow-up appointment. He remarked that her "dog ears," the corners of the large incision, had been diminished to half their size.

My experience has shown that FDM manipulations can have a positive effect on scars in various locations, and the beneficial results are not limited to the aftermath of breast cancer surgery.

Kidney Stones

For the most part, the Fascial Distortion Model is used to address problems that arise from injuries or surgeries, but there are also relevant applications of manipulation techniques for other bodily disorders. One example is the possibility of relieving pain from kidney stones.

The idea is that the ureter, the tube that flows from the kidney to the bladder, may become kinked from the overly tense fascia that surrounds it behind the backbone. Such a kink could block the flow of the kidney stone through the ureter, thereby causing pain. In such a case, the ureter may be unkinked by relieving the tense fascia in the back. Then the stone can pass more easily, and bring more rapid relief from the accompanying pain. The FDM cannot get rid of the stone itself, but it may be able to lessen the pain.

Everything Is Connected

Because the fascia is so interconnected throughout your body, you can get some amazing tensions that become built up and twisted in remote areas. Sometimes in treatment the results seem disconnected from the issue at hand.

For example, I had a man come in for back pain recently, but he also had an irregular heartbeat. He told me "I think they are connected."

"I don't know how that could be," I said.

So we treated his back pain; he felt relieved and went home. When he came back he said, "My back pain is great, and my heart has been regular since you treated me."

"Okay," I said. "That's weird, but I cannot explain it."

Who knows whether there was a connection or it was a mere coincidence? All I can think of is that perhaps his treatment loosened fascia that was affecting a nerve that feeds the heart and generates the heartbeat. Maybe the distorted fascia was causing a kink in the nerve and when I treated him, he went back into a regular rhythm. You can get some pretty interesting things happening in the body.

Another time I treated the pectoral muscle on a woman's chest, and when I pushed above the breast area, it was like somebody snapped a tarp all the way across her chest to her right hip. Everything is connected. We are at the frontiers of research into the many roles that fascia plays in human physiology and we have much to learn. What is clear to me, and what I hope is becoming obvious to the reader, is that with the FDM approach, we are making a major step forward in effectively treating all kinds of musculoskeletal pain.

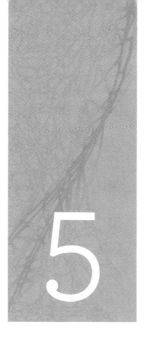

The Model Applied: Treating Injuries Typical of High-Performance Athletes

An incredibly powerful area for the application of Fascial Distortion Model techniques is for high-performance athletes and others who depend on their bodies to accomplish their goals, such as soldiers, dancers, and other performers. From the perspective of the FDM, many of the injuries suffered by these people—especially sprains—can be resolved in minutes. Outside the FDM, as we have seen, such injuries can last for weeks and months before these performers can resume full activity.

As my practice transitioned to full-time osteopathic manipulation, I had the pleasure of seeing an increasing number of athletes as patients. I really enjoy working with those generally striving to reach a higher level of performance. I have worked with runners (from sprinters to ultramarathoners), swimmers, gymnasts, hockey players, and dancers. All of these athletes are pushing themselves toward improving their performance. I have had the honor of treating numerous members of the military (including Navy SEALs, pilots, airborne infantry, and members of Stryker units). Many of these individuals develop distortions and need treatment so they are not sidelined in their pursuit of personal excellence in their careers.

I feel that a solid foundation in the model is critical for the treatment of high-performance athletes. As a provider, I am able to use my clinical experience and understanding to address the limitations these athletes face. I interpret their limitations, listen to their description of the issues, and apply the model to their problems. My treatments are directed at correcting the underlying distortions, which will allow them to have an improved range of movement, decreased pain, and overall improvement in performance.

Once identified, the treatment of their distortions is the same for all of my patients. But interestingly, I have noticed that the body language described by performance athletes can be somewhat vague. These athletes don't emphasize their pain, unless of course I am addressing a specific injury. They speak of their decreased ability. So when I ask a runner, "Where does it hurt?" he or she will often say, "It isn't really pain, but I feel that I can't do this or that. . ." This makes using the physical body language or gestures a little more challenging.

In this chapter, we will examine a variety of injuries that typically plague high-performance athletes.

Shoulders of Swimmers

I have treated a number of swimmers, who commonly suffer from shoulder pain. Traditional medicine tends to focus on the function of the rotator cuff, but I have found that conventional orthopedic treatment of the rotator cuff has not been successful in alleviating the swimmers' pain. I believe that is because much of the shoulder pain is not directly related to rotator cuff injuries. From the FDM perspective, ongoing shoulder pain is consistent with continuum distortions, herniated triggerpoints, and trigger-bands. Foldings of the shoulders are also common. Multiple swimmer patients with prolonged discomfort in the shoulders have responded very well to FDM manipulations.

An Olympic Hopeful

A fourteen-year-old competitive swimmer came to see me because of severe shoulder pain. It was centered in the lateral aspect of the shoulder, near the point of the shoulder (along the subacromial line). She was under quite a bit of stress because she had ambitions to compete in the Olympic Games; on top of that, she was anxious and frustrated because her athletic trainer decided she ought to not use her arms until her shoulder pain got better. She was allowed to go in the pool and kick her legs, but she couldn't actually practice swimming without using her arms. As a rule, this kind of restriction of an athlete's usual performance can be psychologically debilitating.

I was able to get her onto my schedule, and in the course of treatment, she experienced an emotional decompression.

The patient started crying almost at first touch. Of course, we had discussed the discomfort associated with treatment, but before I could work on her shoulder, she basically had an emotional catharsis.

While she regained her composure, I was able to apply the painful FDM technique on her shoulder. The treatment was successful. It took away her pain and restored her range of movement. However, that success sparked a further emotional release and she cried for several hours following the treatment.

I instructed her to resume her pool work and use her arms as tolerated. She continued to improve and did well. Later I learned that, the next day, she participated in the preliminary trials of a swim event. The following week, she went on to win the swim meet. I had not realized she was to participate in the race. I felt a sense of accomplishment after learning that, after being treated, she was immediately able to function at a highly competitive level.

A Runner's Thigh and Knee

Another patient was a runner in training for the Boston Marathon, which was only two weeks away when he came to see me. (This was several years before the tragic bombing.) He came to me despite a strong skepticism that I could help him. He hardly talked at all, but indicated his problem by going up and down his thigh with a flat hand. He said it hurt along the side, and then pointed out two triggerbands below the knee, in the area of his patellar tendon. I couldn't believe how thick this tendon was; it felt like an Achilles tendon.

When I started to treat it, I was amazed to discover about twenty-five triggerbands along the tendon!

What I believe happened is that he tried to cram all his preparation for the Boston Marathon into Alaska's ultra-short running season—about two months before the race. His goal was to run the marathon in less than three hours, so he kept training even as his patellar tendon started thickening. The treatment was successful, and he went on to Boston but missed his goal by four minutes. Highly competitive people like him have no problem working through the pain, and they only slow down when the range of motion gets impaired.

A Soccer Player's Thigh

A soccer player came to me with one of the largest herniated triggerpoints I've ever seen. She stopped suddenly during a game and developed anterior thigh pain and what appeared to be a lump in the muscle. The bulging lump was nearly five inches long. Apparently, the force of her sudden stop had caused a big tear in the fascia on the front of her thigh, and the underlying tissue of the quadriceps muscle moved through the tear. Initially I was worried that she had torn the muscle. The treatment consisted of me basically pushing it all back through the tear and then ironing out the triggerband. She was then able to walk on the leg, and she had full strength. She played soccer ten days later. During that game, a smaller amount of tissue pushed out again so I pushed it back in. She was able to remain active but she elected to take some time off of soccer. Her thigh is now almost back to normal.

A Hockey Player's Ankle

A sixteen-year-old hockey player came to see me on crutches, accompanied by his mother. He had sprained his ankle in a game four days earlier. Another player had collided with him, sending him falling backward over his ankle. He was unable to skate or bear weight on the foot. X-rays indicated no fracture, and in the exam room he showed me his large, purple, swollen foot and ankle.

I told him that the treatment would likely cause a fair amount of discomfort but would last for a very short period of time. He was willing to try it because his team had a big tournament coming up the following week and he wanted to play. I performed a simple treatment of his triggerbands and continuum distortions, plus a single folding treatment. He was then able to walk on the foot, and had regained nearly his full range of motion. It seemed that the swelling was also dramatically reduced, so I asked his mother what she thought. She said the swelling was half as big as it had been when they came into the clinic.

The young man did go off to his hockey tournament; however, he was unable to skate the following weekend because the boot of his skate pressed right on the area of his bruise from the injury. He resumed skating the following week and continued to play hockey with no further difficulty.

In my previous training, I would have had no cure for that ankle. I would have simply told him to put ice on it, use the crutches, and stay away from hockey for a while.

A Cheerleading Gymnastics Instructor with Wrist Pain

I was treating a cheerleading gymnastics instructor for low back pain, which was fairly easily resolved, but then she brought up a problem with her wrists. For several months, her wrists had been sore and weak. She found it very difficult to do a simple push-up without point-tender pain on the side of her wrist. Each time she described the pain she indicated a single spot on her wrist. She had tried physical therapy and had been on multiple anti-inflammatory medications, but these efforts showed no results. We discussed the Fascial Distortion Model and what may be causing this pain. I was able to treat the continuum distortions and resolve the discomfort in her wrist with one or two treatments, to the point that she could do a full push-up without restriction.

A Ballerina's Ankle

A sixteen-year-old ballerina, who was one of the star performers in the local ballet company, came to me with a sprained ankle. We discussed the issues associated with treating the ankle and the fact that it would be painful. I treated multiple triggerbands and continuum distortions in her ankle. She was able to tolerate the treatment quite well and her ankle regained its strength and range of motion. She was able to resume her training for the *Nutcracker* gala performance, and was doing very well.

My daughter also danced in the performance, so in between shows following a matinee, I went backstage to pick her up. I noticed my patient clutching her ankle. My heart sank as I watched this young dancer with tears in her eyes. Then her mother told me that it was the other ankle that hurt, not the one I had treated. Somewhat relieved that she didn't have a relapse, we looked at our next option. I removed an elastic bandage that had been holding an ice pack in place and asked her to move the ankle and show me where her pain was. She was unable to bear weight fully and indicated that any movement at all caused her pain.

Her body language indicated a triggerband, continuum distortions, and a folding in the ankle. I treated these and asked her to show me her range of motion (ROM). Her full ROM had been restored and she was able to go up on pointe without any pain or discomfort. She was essentially back to full function. We wrapped her ankle and applied ice, and she was able to perform in the evening performance without any residual pain or difficulty.

A Dancer's Dislocated Kneecap (Patella)

One week before her company's main performance, a fourteen-year-old ballerina dislocated her kneecap during ballet class. She lost her balance during a routine stretch and twisted her leg, dislocating the kneecap as she fell to the ground. She was unable to bend the knee due to pain, so she was taken to the emergency room over an hour away. She was evaluated in the ER and had to have the patella reduced (put back in position). An orthopedist recommended crutches for up to ten days and suggested a rehabilitation program that could take three to six weeks.

I was able to see her within twenty-four hours of the injury. She could barely bend her knee at all and could not extend it, plus she was in moderately severe pain. Her body language indicated triggerbands going up both sides of the knee along with two continuum distortions just below the kneecap. Treatment of these triggerbands and continuum distortions immediately resulted in full range of movement of the knee. She had some minor stiffness the next day, and was able to dance in the company's performance that weekend without pain.

The u-shaped line identifies the triggerband; the red spots identify the continuum distortions.

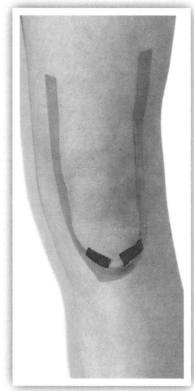

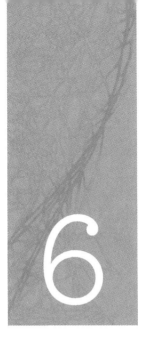

FAQ about Fascia and FDM Treatment

Because the Fascial Distortion Model is a relatively new approach to musculoskeletal pain, many people have questions about fascia and FDM treatments. In this chapter we shall address some of those frequently asked questions.

How can I prepare for an FDM treatment?

When you see a provider who works in the FDM, you should be ready to describe your pain. The provider will ask you to show "where it hurts" and "how it hurts." This is your homework assignment. I want you to remember where and how it hurts. I will even encourage patients to write down their symptoms and locations. Some patients who only experience pain with activity will actually mark places on their body that they would like me to address. They will write on their skin with a pen or marker to identify their areas of pain.

Your verbal explanation of your pain, plus your body language and gestures, should give enough information to practitioners to allow them to diagnose the nature of your fascial distortion. Then they can carry out a treatment directed at the fascia to try to reverse the distortion.

Also we prefer that you apply no heat to the injury for forty-eight hours before the treatment. The only distortion that benefits from heat is a tectonic fixation. For the first treatment we will likely need to address various distortions, and the application of heat could make resolving these problems more difficult.

How painful is the treatment?

There is no getting around the fact that many of the treatments can be quite painful. Treatments typically require a fair amount of force, and that force is most commonly applied with the thumb. Even when I tell patients to brace themselves for pain, it is sometimes stronger than they imagined. The intensity of this pain can cause a person to become nauseated or light-headed, or even break into a cold sweat. Experienced FDM practitioners can often minimize the discomfort by perfecting their own technique. I have found that with practice I am able to improve my ability to gauge the distortion accurately with my thumb, and thereby only apply as much force as is needed to correct the problem.

It is important to remember that not all of the distortions require a painful treatment to be addressed. For example, folding distortions should not really hurt when treated. I do want my patients to understand that some of the treatments are uncomfortable but not everything I do hurts.

What are the side effects?

The primary side effects are bruises and transient tenderness.

Treatments are liable to leave vivid bruises that are dark purple in color. Some of these bruises may last for a long time, and occasionally there are areas of permanent tissue discoloration.

After treatment the affected area can be very tender, but this usually goes away in a day or two. On occasion, the pain following a treatment may last a week or more. Fortunately, this is not usually the case. Despite the tenderness following treatment, I invariably prescribe exercise or some type of movement, even if it is only walking. Movement is good for fascia, and it heals more quickly when your body is in motion.

Do FDM treatments always work?

No. The vast majority of my patients improve with treatment, but not 100 percent. Because the treatments are painful, if my patients did not improve I would have quickly lost interest in this model. It is the overwhelming success of the FDM's results that has encouraged me to devote so much energy to it.

Unfortunately, some patients do not receive benefit from the treatment, and there are several reasons for this:

1. An incorrect diagnosis of the distortion believed to cause the pain.

2. Inadequate treatment. Some FDM practitioners may not have full confidence in the model or in their abilities. In such cases, they may not carry the treatment out completely, which can result in a pain worse than the original complaint. Gaining confidence in the model and in one's skills is a key to providing patients' relief.

3. There can be an underlying issue that is causing the pain other than a fascial distortion.

How can I prevent my fascial distortion from happening again?

I don't know. We have theories and thoughts regarding cause and effect in regard to the distortions, but not enough is known about fascia. It is one of the frontiers of modern medical research. Sometimes distortions just happen.

Is there anything I can do to maintain healthy fascia?

Yes. The quick answer is to maintain an active lifestyle and avoid being sedentary; drink plenty of water; and don't smoke.

Physical activity is a key to our long-term health. It has been said that a sedentary life style is this generation's smoking. The negative health effects associated with our physical inactivity is similar to those if we smoked cigarettes. Physical inactivity is a major health risk. The most basic activity a person can do to benefit their health is to walk. I encourage all of my patients to walk thirty to sixty minutes every day. That should be your goal. A lot of research has shown that walking daily can improve your health.

I feel that even transient inactivity can cause a lot of distortions. Long car rides or airplane flights seem to cause some of the distortions. Sitting at one's desk at work for prolonged periods without a break or a change in position can cause distortions. As silly as it sounds, sleeping in one position can induce certain distortions. It seems our bodies require motion to maintain optimum function.

Another recommendation is hydration. Drinking water is important in the maintenance of our fascial fluidity because fascia is 68 percent water. If we allow ourselves to become relatively dehydrated, this seems to allow distortions to occur more readily.

It appears that the combination of inactivity and dehydration is a very powerful trigger for distortion development. I encourage all of my patients to keep moving and to drink lots of water.

Also, do not smoke! Smoking dries the body out and that is a huge problem. A lot of my back pain patients are smokers.

Do you recommend any activities beyond walking?

Specific types of activities good for your fascia include Pilates, yoga, Tai Chi, and gentle stretching. I recommend slow stretching as opposed to the dynamic stretching where you are bouncing. I will have patients in nursing homes do some long, slow stretches that are not traumatic. Dance and ballet are also good. Perform any activity that encourages your fascial layers to slide and glide on one another. These different exercise regimens all help to keep the tissues moving. Remember, we practitioners do not fix anything; we just get the fascia in the position so the body can fix itself.

Is there any special diet I should follow?

There are many ways to eat healthy. A good start is to increase your vegetable intake and decrease your meat consumption. It is important to decrease the amount of sugar and refined grains in our diet. Good information is available from many resources. I have found diet suggestions from Dr. Andrew Weil to be helpful for patients. Fish oil supplementation and vitamin D appear to be helpful. I recommend patients discuss this with their primary care providers to determine if supplementation is right for them.

Is heat helpful for fascial distortions?

No! Use ice instead. My opinion is that heat bakes fascia together and prevents the slide and glide it needs. Heat seems to temporarily relieve pain, but as soon as the heat is gone and you move, the pain is worse than ever. Heat does feel good sometimes if you have gone on a run and have sore muscles. In that case getting in a hot tub helps work things out, but as a treatment for chronic pain, *heat is not effective.* That's why I encourage ice.

One distortion does respond to heat and that is a tectonic fixation. An example of a tectonic fixation is a frozen shoulder. Heat and gentle stretching could be applied in a situation like this in order to increase the fluidity of the joint lubricant some time prior to treatment.

Do you recommend pain medications?

No. Part of the osteopathic viewpoint is to emphasize physical manipulations instead of medications, and I agree with that. Besides, I honestly think that a lot of fascial pain does not respond well even to narcotic painkillers. My goal in the FDM treatments is to provide pain relief without having to use narcotics. What I've found, having had distortions and treated distortions, is that you can pour narcotics into people all day long and it doesn't do any good. If patients feel they need Advil or Aleve to deal with the tenderness following a treatment, I think that's okay. I don't think such NSAIDs (nonsteroidal anti-inflammatory drugs) are truly necessary, however, because I believe that the mild inflammation has a role to play in the body's overall functions.

However, patients who have been taking narcotic pain-killers for chronic pain for a number of years should not stop cold turkey. They need to talk to their primary physicians and wean off of them gradually. If I have a patient taking narcotics, I will call the primary and say, "The patient is ready to decrease the dosage."

How does the FDM relate to other manipulative or soft tissue approaches, such as massage, chiropractic, physical therapy, rolfing, or acupuncture?

The FDM is a good companion to these modalities. Many of them are also focused on maintaining the body's normal function. I will address them one at a time.

Massage

I strongly support the use of massage to help maintain physical health and fascial movement. Massage in general is a very good way to encourage tissue mobilization. Massage and FDM used together can be very powerful, especially if the massage therapist has an understanding of the FDM. By understanding the distortions and the importance of encouraging and maintaining fascial movement, a massage therapist can often decrease the number of visits to the FDM practitioner.

Of course, there are many styles of massage. Some forms can be very aggressive and deep, but the force of such massage techniques is often applied differently than the forces used in the FDM. In general, I recommend massage once or twice a month as a way to try to reduce the number of visits to my clinic.

Chiropractic

I believe that chiropractic can be most effective when it is done in conjunction with the FDM. Early in my career as an osteopathic physician, I performed some manipulations similar to those performed in the chiropractic arena. They can be quite useful in returning the spine to its proper alignment, but unless you deal with the tensegrity of the fascia that keeps pulling these bones out of alignment, you will only get temporary relief. Thus you have the phenomenon of people making a series of return trips to the chiropractor to keep realigning the spine. If the underlying fascial distortions are corrected, then the alignment issues addressed by chiropractic treatment may be much more lasting.

Physical Therapy

It is very difficult to make a generalization about the effect of combining the FDM with physical therapy (PT), because it is such a diverse field. The ideal situation for such compatibility is when the physical therapist has some understanding and appreciation of the role of fascia in the body. If PT is done with the FDM in mind, it can contribute greatly to a patient's recovery. I have seen the benefits of this a number of times with my patients. However, some physical therapists tend to focus only on the rehabilitation of weak muscles or body structures, and avoid manipulative techniques. Many times, in fact, the tissue perceived by a therapist to be weak or causing an issue becomes stronger and functions normally when the fascial distortion is addressed. This can reduce the amount of time needed for a PT to help a patient reach treatment goals.

Rolfing (Structural Integration)

The use of these techniques together can be powerful. Structural Integration, popularly known as Rolfing, is a manual therapy that is also very concerned about the function of fascia. My understanding is that the technique mobilizes the fascia to restore its motion and function within the body to achieve fluid body mechanics. I've had many patients who have been treated with Rolfing and I've had several patients who work as Rolfers. When speaking with these patients about the theoretical function of the fascia and how it impacts health and musculoskeletal pain, we seem to be on the same page. The main difference I see is that the FDM includes several additional types of distortions that explain fascial function, which are not necessarily addressed in Structural Integration.

Acupuncture

I find acupuncture to be quite complementary to the FDM. The combination of these techniques is often synergistic. The effect of acupuncture on the tissues often helps me address the underlying distortions. Patients who have been treated with acupuncture are often able to more clearly identify troubling distortions. As with physical therapy, not all acupuncturists are created the same. It is good to have a basic understanding as to what type of training and treatments an acupuncture provider uses. Overall, I have referred many patients for acupuncture treatments.

In my opinion as an osteopathic physician, the goal of all these therapies and various treatment styles should be either maintenance of or the rapid return to symmetrical motion. If symmetrical motion is achieved and maintained, then a patient is able to maintain optimum health.

What is the biggest surprise you have encountered when dealing with patients seeking FDM treatments?

My biggest surprise is that people who have lost a lot of weight seem to have an increased tendency to develop distortions. I would have thought it would be the other way around—that overweight patients would be more likely to have distortions. My thought was that the amount of fat in the layers of our fascia would cause problems and allow distortions to occur more readily.

I began asking my patients if they had recently lost or gained weight. I fully expected the answer to be that they had gained weight and then the issues developed. To my surprise, the more common answer was that they had lost weight. I cannot explain this phenomenon.

Perhaps when weight is lost and the fat globules shrink, the fascia is in a relaxed state and more easily distorted. Another thought is that, with weight loss, the body's inflammatory markers (such as TNF-alpha) increase. Could weight loss trigger an inflammatory process in our bodies that makes us more likely to develop distortions? I'm afraid I have more questions than sound theories.

It's important to warn people who have lost as little as ten pounds of weight about the possibility of increased musculoskeletal pain. I have seen many people who successfully lost weight become discouraged due to these unforeseen problems. These are people working hard through diet and exercise to effect a positive health change. Then they are left with musculoskeletal aches and pains that they did not have when they were heavier (sometimes dramatically heavier). If we provide them the counsel that this can occur, they may be more prepared for these changes and more willing to work through the discomfort. We want to provide these people with all the tools to help achieve a better state of health.

The Future of the FDM

All truth passes through three stages.
First, it is ridiculed. Second, it is violently opposed.
Third, it is accepted as being self-evident.

—ARTHUR SCHOPENHAUER, GERMAN PHILOSOPHER

Fasciatopia

In an ideal world as I envision it, every physician in the country would learn the Fascial Distortion Model theory and manipulations as part of their first-and second-year curriculum at medical school. They would be trained to look at the functionality of the human body in a new way: a paradigm that incorporates the dynamic role that fascia plays in facilitating movement, sending pain signals when it becomes distorted, and forming an interconnected matrix throughout the body. The chapters on sprains, sciatica, tennis elbow, and musculoskeletal pain in general would be rewritten to indicate that many of these minor injuries can often be quickly fixed with simple methods at very low cost. Footnotes would warn these students to ignore earlier versions of the textbook that mistakenly said that all injuries such as sprained ankles would take six weeks or more to heal. Professors would chuckle and wonder aloud how anyone could have ever believed such utter nonsense. Those outdated ideas would be relegated to the dustbin of science, along with alchemy, bloodletting, and phlogiston.

Physicians adept at FDM manipulation would be found in every clinic and hospital. Every sports team would have an FDM practitioner, as would every school, every dance company, and every military unit. Billions of dollars would be shaved off the national cost of health care each year, sales of crutches would drop dramatically, and prescriptions for narcotic pain medications would plummet. Most importantly, hundreds of thousands of people—perhaps more—would lead more active lives, free of pain and the tenacious debilitating pull of distorted fascia. If the FDM were embraced by the scientific community and the medical establishment, the world would be a happier, healthier, and wealthier place.

Small Steps

This vision of the future is not merely a grandiose dream. The first small steps toward it have already taken place. We are conducting training courses throughout the year, and several of the instructors routinely have students accompany them in their practices. Some of the greatest experiences I have spreading the model are when working with medical students—who happen to be osteopathic medical students. I work closely with students who get immersed in everyday cases while we treat patients. The advantage of the apprentice-style training portion of the American medical system is that students learn from practicing physicians while treating actual patients. When a medical student sees how quickly a sprained ankle can be treated, that success is indelibly etched in his or her mind, because nothing is more persuasive than firsthand experience. In the future when these students analyze a sprained ankle, they will see fascial distortion as one of the likely diagnoses. They will not blindly accept the traditional view that a sprain is going to take six weeks to heal. Their acceptance is often deep-seated. One student so taken by the results of our treatments asked me, "Why do you need a model? It just is." When learning the Fascial Distortion Model early in one's career, it is hard to consider the body without keeping in mind the importance of fascia.

I am the first to admit that the accomplishments of FDM techniques are hard to believe until you experience them. After all, my introduction to the FDM was as an impromptu patient in between sessions at a medical conference. I didn't read about "miracle cures"; I received one. Two years of pain from my tennis elbows disappeared overnight. That's why I took the FDM seriously. I saw how effective it was for treating patients for everything from recent injuries to chronic conditions lasting more than fifty years. My strong advocacy for the FDM is based on the experience of successfully treating thousands of patients.

Likewise, the awareness of the method among patients is largely spread through word of mouth. Athletes who have experienced the success of the treatments have urged their coaches to provide practitioners to serve their entire teams. Some athletes at a local university are begging their coaches to embrace the FDM. However, the decision-makers at this high level of athletic performance are slow to accept the FDM because it is such a new model. As more people become aware of the theories and implications of the FDM, athletes of all types and levels are appreciating the powerful performance-restoring benefits of it. With each successful treatment, coaches, trainers, and sports medicine physicians are becoming more convinced of its benefits.

Recently, a basketball team in Idaho had a couple of FDM practitioners on the sidelines to treat any injuries that occurred during the game. To my knowledge, that was a first in the United States. Germany is ahead of us in that respect—when a player on the German national soccer team is injured during a game, you see two people in white run onto the field to address the man down. The first is a physician and the second is an FDM practitioner. Once cleared by the physician, the FDM practitioner will actually treat the injured player right on the field and often get him up and running again. In regard to using the model with sports teams, I have no doubt that the competitive spirit is on our side. How would you feel if the opposing team was able to get their injured players back into the game right away while your injured players were given crutches and an ice pack and told to sit out the next few games?

How Do We Get There from Here?

A small but dedicated group of individuals are working to spread the FDM through the American Fascial Distortion Model Association (AFDMA). Recently we were awarded the ability to grant continuing medical education (CME) credit through the American Osteopathic Association (AOA). Our organization also uses the American Association of Family Practice (AAFP) to provide educational courses to physicians, both MDs and DOs. Currently we do not have the system in place to train physical therapists in the FDM. I anticipate that as the organization grows, we will be looking to our colleagues in the physical therapy realm to help treat the legions of patients in need.

In Europe and other countries practitioners other than physicians have been trained in the model. In fact non-physicians make up the largest part of FDM practitioners in those nations. The German FDM practitioner who treats the national soccer team is a physical therapist, not a physician. Each nation has its own laws and customs concerning medical care and licensure; in Germany various practitioners, including physical therapists, are taught to use the model, as well as physicians. In the United States, we have focused on training physicians. This is in part due to limited faculty, and in part related to the hierarchy of medicine here. Our current medical establishment is hesitant to accept new ideas based on anecdotal observations from physicians.

I feel it is important to stress that this is a medical model, because there are serious medical issues that can masquerade as simple distortions. Failure to recognize the underlying medical issues a person may be experiencing could have serious implications. Although the FDM techniques are simple and easy to learn, it is nevertheless a *medical* model that requires a medical perspective. In my practice I am routinely reminding myself to look at the whole person. Recently I had an eighty-year-old woman with chest pain come into my office. My immediate concern was that this was related to her heart. That kind of response is second nature to me because of my years of working as a primary care physician at a walk-in clinic. Fortunately, she was able to tell me the pain had been happening for nearly ten years and that she had been evaluated and treated by a cardiologist and her primary care physician. She had even undergone three cardiac catheterizations for this pain; all were reported as normal. With that information, I was convinced that her issue indeed could be musculoskeletal, and only then did I treat her using the FDM. I was happy that we were able to give her some relief. However, the point is that the FDM is a powerful tool but needs to be used as part of the whole medical system. Maslow's adage comes to mind: "If all you have is a hammer, everything looks like a nail."

Another example of the need to respect the medical context of the model is shown in an experience I had on an international trip with some FDM practitioners. We traveled in Austria with many FDM enthusiasts, only a small portion of whom were physicians. During our free time we hiked to a nearby park, which had a really impressive slide. My daughter went down on it, lost control, hit her head hard on the edge, and shot off the end very shaken. Before we could warn people about the potential danger, one of the FDM practitioners started down the slide. He went down quite rapidly, shot right off the end of it, and landed hard on his ankle. Quickly a crowd gathered, and being FDM practitioners, started treating the distortions on his ankle that were identified by the patient. I was immediately concerned that he may have broken the ankle and tried to warn them: "I think he *broke* his ankle! You may want to stabilize it and get an x-ray." As a physician, I had been trained to evaluate injured ankles using the Ottawa criteria to determine whether it might be broken. But the others could not be distracted from the patient showing them distortions, so they kept trying to treat it. Several days later, the man ended up going to surgery to have nine screws placed in his ankle. . . because it was *broken*. We cannot ignore the medical diagnoses that accompany the distortions.

As our organization grows, I anticipate we will have a process in place to train our physical therapy colleagues in the theory and techniques of the FDM. I look forward to working with them to help our mutual patients heal faster and regain activity sooner.

Courting the Establishment

Our master plan for bringing the Fascial Distortion Model to the masses requires gaining the acceptance of the medical establishment. It is very difficult for any new ideas to be embraced, especially since we live in an era of evidence-based research. I always find this mindset kind of interesting because new ideas and thoughts are held to a standard that the old theories can't meet. We cannot go back in time and find the evidence for a lot of our treatments, but if there is anything new, it now needs to be supported by evidence-based research. Research is very expensive—especially in a clinical setting where there is not typically enough financial support to carry out a research program. But research will no doubt be helpful in convincing the naysayers of the truth of the FDM, and that is one crucial element we need for it to go forward.

A place the FDM will likely find support is within the establishment of osteopathic medicine, and there are two reasons for that. The first is that the FDM helps to explain the overall osteopathic paradigm, which holds that everything in the body is connected. We believe that fascia is the ultimate interconnective tissue in the body. Understanding the overarching importance of fascia and its biotensegrital structure would support and extend the osteopathic perspective. This attitude was shared by several key leaders of the American Academy of Osteopathy who sat through some of my weekend seminars on the FDM. They said this model explains osteopathy. The FDM is clearly a new way of looking at the body that fits into the osteopathic model of interconnectedness.

The other reason to encourage osteopathic medicine to embrace the FDM is its tradition of manipulation, even though the use of manipulation by DOs needs to be revitalized in practice. Osteopaths are taught a lot of different styles of manipulation as part of their medical school curriculum. We learn techniques ranging from high-velocity, low-amplitude articulation (HVLA) of the vertebrae and bones, which many people associate with chiropractic, to more soft tissue techniques, including cranial sacral, balanced ligamentous tension, fascial unwinding, and facilitated positional release. Osteopathy includes a diverse collection of different techniques used to achieve the physiological goal of symmetrical motion. However, we do not want the FDM to be seen as just another technique or style. We want it to be recognized for its emphasis on the inherent importance of fascia in general. In this way, we are trying to reintroduce the importance of fascia into osteopathic medicine and all medicine.

The mindset of the mainstream medical establishment also presents challenges. I was invited to present a training seminar at a major medical facility in the Midwest, but they hesitated to have me attend because our current direction was to only train physicians. The administrators wanted to include physical therapists, because they felt that MDs would be averse to learning hands-on techniques. This sense of hierarchy in the medical profession carries a catch-22. Some MDs may feel that physical manipulation is beneath them, but at the same time, they are not likely to be persuaded of the value of the FDM by a physical therapist. Not all physicians value the skills that our physical therapy colleagues possess. Even as a physician myself, I often have a tough time persuading my fellow physicians of the value of my work.

The Money Factor

One thing that everyone can agree on is that our healthcare system is too darn expensive. I'm sick of seeing surveys that indicate the United States spends more on health care per capita than any other developed country, yet shows poorer results. That has to be one of the best reasons to spread the practice of the FDM, a low-cost treatment with fantastic results.

The Affordable Care Act and the cost of health care has been a hot topic of conversation and debate for years. The rapidly rising cost of health care has reached a critical point. As we look forward, we see the incredible financial burden that health care will have on our economy. The numbers associated with musculoskeletal pain and treatment are astounding. A simple solution that would save billions of dollars would be to train all physicians to use the FDM in their diagnoses. This would save money in three ways:

1. **Preventing erroneous diagnoses**, thus preventing expensive treatment that doesn't work. It is not unusual for patients to undergo expensive diagnostic testing or prolonged physical therapy, and be prescribed multiple medications for conditions that may be actually related to an easily remedied fascial distortion. Here are some examples:

   - **Sciatica**: To most minds, every pain in a butt cheek that radiates down the leg is sciatica. But in reality, only about 10 percent of the people who think they have sciatica actually have it. The remaining 90 percent often have some sort of fascial distortion, usually a herniated triggerpoint.

   - **Tennis elbow**: This is a great example, because everybody knows that tennis elbow is inflammation—that's what we're taught in medical school. So over the past twenty-five years, we've always treated tennis elbow as inflammation. We will give anti-inflammatory medicine; we will give steroid injections; we will even use ice and physical therapy. All of these treatments are geared toward trying to reduce inflammation. An MRI often does not show inflammation, yet that's what we treat. But if you treat a sprained elbow or tennis elbow with the FDM and the pain is gone immediately, then obviously it was not due to inflammation.

- **Abdominal pain**: A woman I treated for abdominal pain had undergone tens of thousands of dollars of treatments and testing. Yet after a simple diagnosis according to the model, we treated her and gave her dramatic relief.

- **Arthritis**: Frequently I will see a person who has been diagnosed with arthritis in the lower back, even though their pain doesn't correlate with the arthritis seen on imaging.

2. **Starting with an inexpensive diagnosis** rather than jumping to expensive tests. Just imagine the cost savings to our health-care system if providers looked at patients in the FDM before ordering MRIs, CT scans, or x-rays. If the FDM doesn't explain and improve their pain, *then* the testing, medications, and other modalities could be tried.

- If I see somebody for back pain, I will treat him or her and say, "If that pain returns within four hours, we may have to do a CT scan to rule out a kidney stone." You do a quick check for fascial distortion before you jump to the big expense of a CT scan. I have treated some people for a couple of weeks and given them some pain relief, but it doesn't last. That's when we end up doing the MRI and finding out whether they have a herniated disc.

- In medicine now it seems that everybody goes directly to the MRI, which costs $1,200 to $1,500, and that is not necessary. Many doctors these days are not comfortable making a complicated diagnosis based on a physical examination. They rely on the imaging and other expensive tests, which increases the cost of care.

3. **Boosting productivity by cutting down on sick days**: Most patients are members of the work force who must take sick days to visit the doctor's office, get tests, and receive physical therapy. Think of the many hours of sick leave, lost productivity, and reduced productivity when they do go to work— all because they have been misdiagnosed and are wasting their time when they could be pain-free and fully functioning.

Perhaps insurance companies can indirectly help the cause of the FDM, because they are always trying to save money on medical treatments. There is a movement called "From Volume to Value" that the insurance industry seems to be spearheading. The idea is to move away from the current system that pays providers based on the volume of services they provide to patients, and toward a payment system based on rewarding providers who achieve results— thus, it is a better value. The insurance companies feel that paying for volume tends to provide an incentive for inefficient treatments—that *more* is not necessarily *better*. While physicians in general may be very apprehensive about this change, this new system would work in favor of physicians using the FDM, because we already are providing efficient treatments. However, our success is not widely known. If the payment for value plan comes into effect, patients could use online search queries like, "Who provides the best value for sprained ankles?" If they search for those who give the best results, I have no doubt that FDM practitioners will get high ratings.

Let the Patient Be Your Guide

I can discuss the medical establishment, insurance companies, and international conferences, but the future growth of the Fascial Distortion Model will really depend on the patients. It was patients who guided the discovery of the FDM, and I believe it will be the patients who will guide it into the future. Each patient who receives a successful FDM treatment becomes an ambassador for the cause, spreading the word of this important new approach to various sorts of musculoskeletal ailments. Their personal testimony to their friends and acquaintances is more valuable than any book or research study.

We all strive for health and happiness in our own way, finding challenges and joys at work, at home, and with our families. My message is a simple one. Moving your body helps you to heal yourself, and my job is to remove the pain and tensions that restrict your full range of symmetrical motion. By helping to enable you to move, you can gain the inner strength you need in life to meet your challenges and appreciate your joys.

It is my hope that this book will enable you to understand the FDM enough so that you will seek it out if you haven't already. Creating a demand for an important service sends a strong message to the powers that be. Individuals making a grassroots effort in pursuit of happiness is the most valuable fruit of our democracy, and I have no doubt that a multitude of your voices will make a powerful difference. Good luck to you all, and keep that fascia moving!

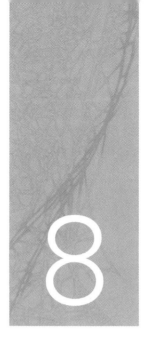

FDM at a Glance

The Fascial Distortion Model (FDM)

Founder: Stephen Typaldos, DO, identified his first distortion—a triggerband—in 1991 when a patient insisted that he press on a pain in her back. In the next few years he developed the Fascial Distortion Model and identified the six basic distortions.

Definition: The FDM is a new approach to how the human body is constructed and how it should be treated for musculoskeletal injuries, side effects of surgery, and various other conditions.

Fascia: The key idea of the FDM is that the fibrous tissues of fascia that form a matrix throughout the body are responsible for the fluid movement of body parts but, when distorted, cause pain and limit the range of movement.

- A key component in the biotensegrity of the body—a moveable structure composed of flexible connectors exerting tension on the bones and soft tissues.

- It is a flexible interface that allows the "slide and glide" of muscles and ligaments.

- Its strength contributes to the movement of the body.

Key Tips for Healthy Fascia:

- Keep it moving (walk, stretch, exercise).

- Drink plenty of water.

- Eat healthy food.

- Don't smoke.

- Don't sit still for too long.

Diagnosis: FDM practitioners diagnose fascial distortions based on the patient's verbal report, body language, and gestures to describe the pain.

Treatments: Fascial distortions are usually treated with manipulations, most often administered by a strong and sensitive thumb. The objective is to undo the distortions and push the fascia back into shape, thus relieving pain and restoring movement.

The Six Basic Distortions:

1) Triggerband (TB): Distorted banded fascial tissue. This is a relatively common type of fascial distortion and is the easiest to repair. It was the first distortion to be identified by Dr. Typaldos.

- **Symptoms**: Burning, pulling, pain along a line.

- **Body Language**: Sweeping motion with fingers along painful linear pathway.

- **Feels Like**: A ribbon or violin string.

- **Treatment**: Use thumb to untwist and iron out the wrinkled tissue.

2) Herniated Triggerpoint (HTP): Abnormal protrusion of tissue through a fascial plane. I see more patients with HTPs than any other distortion.

- **Symptoms**: An ache, pinching, or catching.

- **Body Language**: Pushes the thumb or fingers into a specific spot.

- **Feels Like**: A knot or a grape.

- **Treatment**: Push the knot back through the hole in the fascia.

3) Continuum Distortion (CD): An alteration of the transition zone between ligament, tendon, other connective tissue and bone.

- **Symptoms**: A specific spot of pain on a bone.

- **Body Language**: Single finger points to a specific spot.

- **Feels Like**: A small grain of rice.

- **Treatment**: Push on the distortion until it shifts, pops, or melts, thus shifting back to neutral.

4) Folding Distortion (FD): A three-dimensional alteration of a fascial plane. It is most often found in a hinge-type joint, such as the wrist, elbow, or shoulder. It can also occur in the areas between muscles and between bones.

- **Symptoms**: Deep ache in the joint that feels like it restricts movement, but when tested the range of motion is normal.

- **Body Language**: Patient cups hands over the joint.

- **Treatment**: Repeat the injury: pull on an unfolding and push on a refolding.

5) Cylinder Distortion (CyD): The overlapping of cylindrical fascial coils. This is the most bizarre, mysterious, and elusive distortion. Providers not using the FDM may suspect the problem is merely psychological.

- **Symptoms**: Bizarre symptoms such as pain that fluctuates or jumps from one area to another, numbness, tingling, tremor, impression of swelling.

- **Body Language**: Hand appears to squeeze or sweep the pain away.

- **Feels like**: Difficult to feel; may have to use a pet comb to find tangle.

- **Treatment**: Untangle fascia coils with hands, cups, pet comb, baby-vac, and so on.

6) Tectonic Fixation (TF): An inability of the fascial surfaces to glide, so they are stuck together. A frozen shoulder is a common example.

- **Symptoms**: Joint that won't move.

- **Body Language**: Grabs joint and tries to jiggle it; tries to move joint with force.

- **Treatment**: Slow pumping of fluid between the layers, followed by joint mobilization; heat may increase fluidity of the joint lubricant.

Fascial Distortion Model (FDM)

FDM is a model of thinking that provides a framework to view the function of the body. Fascia is the "wrapper" of our bones, muscles and organs, and is an integral part of the body's nerve network. Treatments in the model focus on restoring the function of fascia by correcting distortions in the system, and thereby eliminating pain.

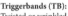

Triggerbands (TB):
Twisted or wrinkled fascial fibers that cause a burning or pulling pain along the course of the fascial band.

Herniated Triggerpoints (HTP):
HTP's are pathological herniations of tissue through a fascial plane. Pain from HTP is often described as a deep ache.

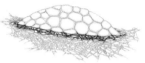

Folding Distortions (FD):
These injuries are similar to what happens to a road map that unfolds and then refolds in a contorted condition. Folding distortions hurt deep in the joint.

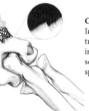

Continuum Distortions (CD):
Injuries of the bone/fascia transition zone. Pain is identified in one spot. These are commonly seen in plantar fasciitis and sprained ankles.

Cylinder Distortions (Cyl):
Anatomically reminiscent of a tangled Slinky® toy, cylinder distortions cause deep pain in predominantly non-jointed areas. They are also responsible for a wide range of seemingly bizarre symptoms, such as tingling (paresthesia), numbness (diminished sensation), and pain that spontaneously seems to jump from one location to another.

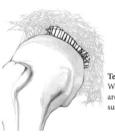

Tectonic Fixations (TF):
When patients complain of joint stiffness, they are describing a tectonic fixation. TF's are fascial surfaces which have lost their ability to glide.

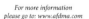

For more information
please go to: www.afdma.com

©2013 AFDMA.
Artwork by Brianna Reagan Art, @2013

This poster is available for sale on the website of the American Fascial Distortion Model Association, **www.afdma.com**

Common Problems Often Addressed Through FDM Manipulations (in alphabetical order):

- Abdominal pain
- Ankle pain
- Back pain
- Frozen shoulder
- Headaches
- Flank pain consistent with kidney stone pain
- Knee pain
- Neck pain
- Pelvic pain
- Plantar fasciitis
- Post-surgery pain
- Rib pain
- Shoulder pain
- Sprained ankles
- Tennis elbow
- Thigh pain
- Wrist pain

About the AFDMA

When Dr. Typaldos suddenly passed away, the growth of the Fascial Distortion Model (FDM) movement in the United States was essentially a rudderless ship. A courageous group of his colleagues, students, and friends formed an organization focused on spreading the FDM in the medical world in an effort to guide the movement. This group is committed to the spread and advancement of the model.

Dr. Typaldos had the goal of seeing the FDM in the hands of every physician.

The mission of the AFDMA is to promote the use of the FDM to diagnose and treat musculoskeletal injuries and medical conditions, by:

1. Informing and educating the medical community about the FDM

2. Establishing certification standards for FDM practitioners and instructors in the United States

3. Providing training and certification for FDM practitioners and instructors

4. Promoting and funding research on the application of the FDM

5. Working in cooperation with the European FDM Association (EFDMA), the FDM Asia Association (FAA), and the African FDM Society (AFDMS) to coordinate standards of certification and training worldwide

6. Informing and educating the public about the FDM

7. Promoting the appropriate use of the FDM by well-trained health professionals in the United States

The AFDMA is a nonprofit corporation approved by the IRS as a 501(c)(3) tax-exempt organization and classified as a public charity. Contributions are tax deductible to the extent permitted by law.

If you are interested in learning more about this organization's activity or would like to purchase posters of the distortions, please visit the website of the American Fascial Distortion Model Association (**www.AFDMA.com**).

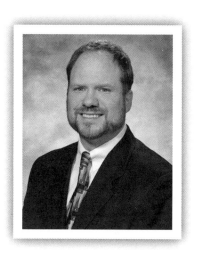

Todd Capistrant, DO

Dr. Todd Capistrant is an osteopathic physician who has increasingly centered his practice on the Fascial Distortion Model. In addition to his busy osteopathic manipulative practice, he currently serves as the Chief Medical Officer for Tanana Valley Clinic/Banner Health in Fairbanks, Alaska. He is a board member of the AFDMA, and routinely engaged as one of its instructors to teach the FDM throughout the world. He also serves as a regional dean for Pacific Northwest University, an osteopathic medical school located in Yakima, Washington, bringing Alaskan osteopathic students back to Fairbanks for training. Todd lives near Denali National Park with his wife and two daughters who maintain a sled dog kennel and farm homestead. Both he and his wife have competed in and finished the Iditarod Trail Sled Dog Race. He and his family enjoy being active outdoors and frequently can be found enjoying outdoor pursuits in Alaska and wherever their travels may take them.

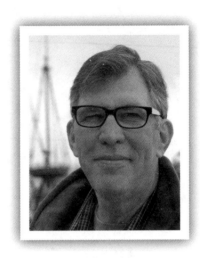

About Steve LeBeau

Steve is a writer and editor based in St. Paul, Minnesota. He is a former journalist and was a speechwriter for Minnesota Governor Jesse Ventura.

Steve can be contacted at **steve@splebeau.com**.

Acknowledgments

In writing this book, I would like to acknowledge the work of Dr. Stephen Typaldos. The Fascial Distortion Model was developed and elucidated in his work and through the publication of his textbooks. His teaching inspired many physicians to a new level of understanding. The genius of his effort is the combination of traditional osteopathic principles and practice with an emphasis placed on the importance of fascial tissue and the distortions that can occur within the body. Through his work we are able to provide patients with relief of their musculoskeletal pain.

I would like to acknowledge and thank my parents, Dr. Terrance and Jacqueline Capistrant, for their encouragement and support to become a physician. Without their guidance I may have never even started down the road toward medical school.

I would like to acknowledge and thank my wife, Anne, and my daughters Rose and Grace. They have had endless patience and provided tremendous support and encouragement. Their love and understanding has allowed me to spend time away from them treating patients and teaching. I am so grateful for the hard work they do keeping our homestead running. Coming home to you is my happiness.

I would like to acknowledge the support of my colleagues in Fairbanks, Alaska. As my practice evolved into one of manual medicine, they were supportive and encouraging in my efforts. Their graciousness has provided me with the opportunity to help our mutual patients by reducing their pain and restoring them to better mobility.

My hat's off to all the physicians, both MDs and DOs, who take the time to train students and further our profession. Without the effort you put into medical education, we would not be able to continue training physicians. To all of my teachers, thank you for your efforts. I would also like to thank all of the osteopathic physicians who paved the way for the DOs of today. Your diligence to our profession allows me to be an osteopathic physician.

Most importantly I would like to thank the patients. As we sought relief of your musculoskeletal complaints, you have allowed me to develop a further understanding of the human body and how to apply that knowledge to help other patients. For this, I am grateful.

Notes

1. J. Hasselström, J. Liu-Palmgren, and G. Rasjö-Wrååk, "Prevalence of pain in general practice," in *European Journal of Pain*, 2002, 6: 375–385. DOI: 10.1016/S1090-3801(02)00025-3.

2. Agency for Healthcare Research and Quality. "Translating Research Into Practice (TRIP)-II: Fact Sheet," March 2001: http://www.ahrq. gov/research/findings/factsheets/translating/tripfac/index.html (retrieved on 01.10.14).

3. Dr. Typaldos told this story on a videotape I watched at a conference in Vienna; it is also recounted in a book by his assistant, Marjorie Kasten, PT, *FDM: An Introduction to the Fascial Distortion Model*, 2010, an AFDMA publication, pp.7-8.

4. Aaron Young, PhD, Humayun J. Chaudhry, DO, MS, Jon V. Thomas, MD, MBA, and Michael Dugan, MBA, "A Census of Actively Licensed Physicians in the United States," in *Journal of Medical Regulation*, Volume 99, Number 2, 2013, p 13.

5. Typaldos, Stephen, DO, *FDM: Clinical and Theoretical Application of the Fascial Distortion Model Within the Practice of Medicine and Surgery*, 2002: Typaldos Publishing Co.

6. Still, A.T. (Andrew Taylor), *Philosophy of Osteopathy*, 1899: http://www.gutenberg.org/files/25864/25864-h/25864-h.htm#Page_11

7. Ingber DE, "The architecture of life," in *Scientific America* 1998 Jan; 278(1): 48-57.

8. Typaldos, *FDM: Clinical and Theoretical Application of the Fascial Distortion Model Within the Practice of Medicine and Surgery*.

9. Ibid.

Index